PROF. ARNOLD EHRET'S
MUCUSLESS DIET
HEALING
SYSTEM

ANNOTATED, REVISED, AND EDITED BY PROF. SPIRA

A SCIENTIFIC METHOD OF EATING YOUR WAY TO HEALTH

PROF. ARNOLD EHRET'S

MUCUSLESS DIET HEALING SYSTEM

ANNOTATED, REVISED, AND EDITED BY PROF. SPIRA

By Prof. Arnold Ehret (1866-1922)

Annotated, Revised, and Edited by Prof. Spira

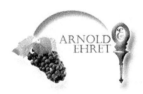

Published by Breathair Publishing

Columbus, OH

2nd Edition 2014

Printed by CreateSpace, an Amazon.com Company
CreateSpace, Charleston SC

Available from www.mucusfreelife.com, Amazon.com, on Kindle, and other retail outlets

Printed in the United States of America

First issued and printed as a Breathair Publishing Paperback, 2014
Second Printing, 2015
Revised, November 2015

Second Edition

ISBN-13: 978-0-9906564-0-1
ISBN-10: 0-9906564-0-3
www.mucusfreelife.com

CONTENTS

BIOGRAPHICAL SKETCH OF PROF. ARNOLD EHRET

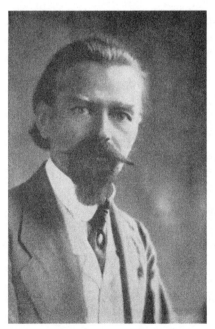

Professor Arnold Ehret was a German healer, dietitian, philosopher, teacher, visionary, and one of the first people to advocate fasting and a plant-based, vegan, and mucus-free lifestyle as a therapy for healing. For over 100 years, his written works and teachings have touched the lives of thousands of health-seekers pursuing higher levels of vitality. Ehret's most famous books, *Mucusless Diet Healing System* and *Rational Fasting*, continue to increase in popularity as plant-based, vegan, and raw-food diets become more prevalent. Ehret believed that pus- and mucus-forming foods were unnatural for humans to eat, and suggested that a diet of fruits and green leafy vegetables (i.e., mucus-free foods), are the most healing and powerful foods for humans. Ehret offers a sophisticated yet simple and safe transitional system for those who endeavor to stop eating pus- and mucus-forming foods.

1

Early Life

Arnold Ehret was born July 29, 1866, near Freiburg, in Baden, Germany. His father was a gifted farmer who was so technologically advanced that he crafted all of his own farming equipment. Like his father, Ehret would be endowed with a passion for studying the cause and effect of phenomena. His courses of interest were physics, chemistry, drawing, and painting. He also had an affinity for linguistics and could speak German, French, Italian, and English.

At the age of 21, he graduated as a professor of drawing and was drafted into the military only to be discharged because of heart trouble. At the age of 31, he was diagnosed with Bright's disease (inflammation of the kidneys) and pronounced incurable by 24 of Europe's most respected doctors. He then explored natural healing and visited sanitariums to learn holistic methods and philosophies. In a desperate attempt to quench his misery, Ehret decided to stop eating. To his amazement, he did not die but gained strength and vitality.

In 1899, he traveled to Berlin to study vegetarianism, followed by a trip to Algiers in northern Africa where he experimented with fasting and fruit dieting. Due to his new lifestyle, Ehret completely cured himself of all of his diseases and could then perform great feats of physiological strength, including an 800-mile bicycle trip from Algiers to Tunis. His discovery caused him to posit that pus- and mucus-forming foods are the fundamental cause for all human illness, and that fasting (simply eating less) is Nature's primary method of cleansing the body of the effects of unnatural eating.

Successful Healer

In the early 1900s, Ehret opened a hugely popular sanitarium in Ascona, Switzerland where he treated and cured thousands of patients considered incurable by the so-called "medical authorities." During the latter part of the decade, Ehret engaged in a series of fasts monitored by German and Swiss officials. Within a period of 14 months, Ehret completed one fast of 21 days, one of 24 days, one of 32 days, and one of 49 days, which stood as a world record for many years. Ultimately, Ehret became one of the most in-demand health lecturers, journalists, and educators in Europe, saving the lives of thousands of people.

On June 27, 1914, just before World War I, Ehret left from Bremen for the United States to see the Panama Exposition and sample the fruits of the continent. He found his way to California, which was of special interest to him. This was because the region was undergoing a horticultural renaissance due to botanists like Luther Burbank, who later paid tribute to Ehret. At the time, the University of California, Riverside also owned the world's largest collection of rare fruits. When the war prevented Ehret from returning to Germany, he settled in Mount Washington (Los Angeles), where he prepared his manuscripts and diplomas in his cultivated eating gardens. He and other "Back to Naturists" began to influence local populations of young people to investigate plant-based, natural living.

Benedict Lust, a student of Ehret's and early proponent of naturopathy, initially distributed the English-language books of Ehret, Kneipp, Kuhne, Just, and Engelhardt in the United States. This included Ehret's *Kranke Menschen* (literally, sick human beings) which became a best seller. Ehret worked at Lust's Yungborn Sanitarium for 5 years. Then, Ehret opened his own sanitarium in Alhambra, California before a lecture tour. His course on the *Mucusless Diet Healing System* became a book of 25 lessons for his students. The book, along with *Rational Fasting*, became his most important and popular publications. Ehret also developed and marketed his popular Innerclean Herbal Laxative formula.

Death

On October 9, 1922, just 2 weeks after he completed the *Mucusless Diet Healing System*, he finished a series of four lectures on regaining health through fasting and the "Grape Cure" (grape and grape juice fasting) at the Assembly Room of the Angelus Hotel on 4th and Spring Streets, where it was reported that over a hundred persons were unable to find seats. After leaving the building, between 11:00 p.m. and 11:30 p.m., Ehret, aged 56, fell and sustained a fatal blow to his skull. According to Ehret's business partner and publisher, Fred S. Hirsch, DNS, he was walking briskly on a wet, oil-soaked street during foggy conditions when he slipped on the curb and fell backward onto his head. Hirsch did not actually witness the fall but found Ehret lying on the street. Carl Kuhn, Ehret's German publisher during the 1920s, even questioned whether Ehret's fall was

3

really an accident. Benedict Lust maintained that Ehret was wearing his first pair of new dress shoes and slipped as a result of his unfamiliarity with the footwear.

To this day, the true nature of Ehret's death raises suspicion among his followers. Ehret's powerful healing successes along with his influential and revolutionary new lifestyle threatened the medical, meat, and dairy industries. Due to these factors, many believe that foul play was involved in Ehret's untimely death. His writings on religion and family were also considered quite controversial. In the decades following Ehret's death, Fred Hirsch had many legal battles with medical authorities over the word "mucus" and the Innerclean laxative.

Legacy

Arnold Ehret is a cultural icon and was an important protagonist of the emerging back-to-nature renaissance in Germany and Switzerland during the latter part of the nineteenth century. The influence of this renaissance spread to America and influenced many counter-cultural movements including the beat generation, the vegetarian-driven "hippie" movement, veganism, and fruitarianism. Throughout the twentieth century, Ehret's teachings have thrived and developed through the sincere efforts of a small group of dedicated Ehretists. Today, Ehret's teachings are gaining wider acceptance throughout the world as more people seek to investigate plant-based, vegan healing and detoxification.

-*Prof. Spira, June 2013*

INTRODUCTION TO THE ANNOTATED VERSION

Greetings Brothers and Sisters,

When I began practicing the *Mucusless Diet Healing System* 13 years ago, I had the privilege of having access to a community of practitioners that had built on Arnold Ehret's profound work and developed it into a sustainable lifestyle and dietetic art form. I spent hours talking with them about the details of the book and had all of my newbie questions thoroughly answered. Brother Air, the 35-year practitioner of the mucusless diet who introduced me to it, took me to supermarkets and showed me how to shop for the diet. He also would invite me into his home to show me how to properly prepare food. My intensive analysis of the *Mucusless Diet Healing System* book, unprecedented access to some of the most advanced practitioners in the world, and more than a decade of experience, have helped me to gain the insights necessary to create the following annotated version. I take little credit for my additions, and must humbly thank Brother Air, Victor B., Khaleeq, and the many others who took the time to help me learn as much about the mucusless diet as possible. I would also like to thank Fred Hirsch, Ehret's most trusted student and most important proliferator of his works, and Alvin Last, who purchased Ehret Publishing from Fred Hirsch in the early 1970s and kept the books in print into the twenty-first century. And of course, I would also like to thank Arnold Ehret, whose genius has changed the lives of multitudes of people.

The inspiration for this newly edited, updated, and annotated version of Arnold Ehret's *Mucusless Diet Healing System* emerged about 2 years after I had read the book. I could not stop reading the book over and over again, and found it to be a true work of genius! Yet, as I began to examine it more deeply, I noticed certain issues that might prevent first-time or contemporary readers from gaining full comprehension. Occasional archaic and hard-to-understand syntax, content contradictions, and the author's collegial attempts to have dietetic dialogs with his peers, all of whom he was miles ahead of, cause many readers to misunderstand some aspects of his message.

Over the years, I have received many of the same questions from *Mucusless Diet* readers. The purpose of this book is to address some of the most common questions and make editorial updates for a twenty-first century audience. My goal is not to rewrite the *Mucusless Diet*, but to create a reference document that will facilitate comprehension and understanding for modern audiences. My notes and additions will appear in several ways, including endnotes, italicized and indented purports before or after lessons, and editorial notes inserted into a chapter. Exceptions include the reworking of the Ragnar Berg's table for clarity, and updates to some of the vegetarian recipes added by the editor Fred Hirsch. Thorough explanations precede all such alterations.

What is the best way to use this book? If you have never read the *Mucusless Diet Healing System* before, I suggest the following method. Read each chapter in its entirety, skipping over all of the notes. Then, immediately reread the chapter with your primary focus being on the annotations. If you are already familiar with Ehret's original work, then the best method for you may be to read the annotations as you go along from the beginning. This document can also be used as a reference book to quickly look up common questions related to the diet.

The principles of the *Mucusless Diet Healing System* are timeless and desperately needed today. In a world where there is much confusion about the nature of human illness, Ehret provides a simple, yet incredibly advanced, system to achieve wellness and superior health.

Peace, Love, and Breath!

-Prof. Spira, September 2015

FOREWORD

We read in the Bible, Genesis 1:29: "I have given you every herb bearing seed which is upon the earth—and every tree in which is the fruit yielding seed; to you it shall be for meat." You will note that the word "meat" is used to denote human's "food," not the carcass of dead animals! Arnold Ehret was a student and follower of Nature's laws—in communion with GOD! Ehret's teachings have their foundation in TRUTH—but until they are "demonstrated," the average individual cannot grasp their significance and consequently—not until then—do they prove acceptable to the great majority!

Arnold Ehret described and denounced superstition and ignorance, but like similar teachings of great men, his teachings have been grossly misunderstood by the average individual and unjustly criticized by many health teachers. It has now been well over 70 years that his voice was first heard vainly sounding a note of warning, desperately hoping to dispel the colossal ignorance of the average uninformed individual concerning Natural laws! His teachings have opened many new avenues of healing, and his wonderful philosophy and knowledge offered to those willing to accept bring thousands of new converts each year, from every part of the globe!

Ehret taught that the mind governs all organic action of the physical body instinctively and we therefore find humankind gradually evolving from the primitive stage to a higher intellectual plane. The physical and mental welfare of millions of individuals

7

living today are desperately searching for a truthful presentation of this knowledge found only in Prof. Arnold Ehret's message and it is therefore eagerly awaited by an expectant world! Is it asking too much that you lay aside preconceived ideas, opinions, or prejudices and read the Ehret articles with an open mind? Hopefully the truth will eventually dawn upon you, possibly months after reading—for some portion may have indelibly stamped an imprint on your mind— and intuitively proven its correctness!

There is no "mystery" connected with Ehret's "Mucusless Diet" theory—though it differs almost entirely from other "healing systems," especially his lucid explanations. Ehret practiced no deception; his statements are easily understood because of their outstanding "simplicity" of expression. He continually informs the student, "Whatsoever is not simple—easily understood, is 'false' and therefore not the truth!"

Fundamentally, Ehret's teachings of his philosophy are basically the love of NATURE itself—love of all outdoors! The love of flowers and trees, the love of all of the birds and animals! Ehret loved the sunshine and the rain, the cold and the warmth, the bright days and the cloudy days. And he sincerely taught that we must feel justly proud of our own physical bodies—CLEAN both internally and externally!

Our "love" of birds and four-legged animals instinctively warns that we must not harm these fellow creatures—and never kill them for our food! Mother Nature has abundantly supplied us with quantities of delicious, nutritious fruits and vegetables on which we thrive! With a clean bloodstream coursing through our bodies, any thought of cannibalism becomes obnoxious.

Arnold Ehret taught tolerance! Respect for the rights of others and acceptance of their rights to their own beliefs! Never attempt to force others to accept your beliefs, but rather through precept and example create a desire on the part of those interested in health to seek this great truth of their own free will! Through your tolerance of "ignorance," you will have proven your superiority, and eventually "nonbelievers" will see the bright glow of TRUTH!

-Fred S. Hirsch, DNS (Ehret Literature)

8

General Introductory Principles

Lesson I

Every disease, no matter what name it is known by medical science, is

Constipation

It is a clogging up of the entire pipe system of the human body.[1] Any special symptom is therefore merely an extraordinary local constipation by more accumulated mucus at this particular place.[2] Special accumulation points are the tongue, the stomach, and particularly the entire digestive tract. This last is the real and deeper cause of bowel constipation. The average person has as much as 10 pounds of uneliminated feces in the bowels, continually poisoning the bloodstream in the entire system.[3] Think of it!

Every sick person has a more or less mucus-clogged system, such mucus being derived from undigested, uneliminated, and unnatural food substances accumulated from childhood on. Details regarding this fact may be learned by reading my *Rational Fasting and Regeneration Diet*.

My "Mucus Theory" and *Mucusless Diet Healing System* stand unshaken; it has proven the most successful "Compensation Action" so-called cure against every kind of disease.[4] By its systematic application, thousands of declared-incurable patients could be saved.

9

The mucusless diet consists of all kinds of raw and cooked fruits, starchless vegetables, and cooked or raw mostly green-leaf vegetables.[5] The *Mucusless Diet Healing System* is a combination of individually advised, long or short fasts with progressively changing menus of *non-Mucus-Forming Foods*. This diet alone can heal every case of "disease" without fasting, although such a cure requires longer time.[6] The system itself will be expounded in later lessons.

However, to learn how to apply this system and understand how and why it works, it is necessary to free your mind of medical errors, partly taken by naturopathy.[7] In other words, I must teach you a new *physiology*, free from medical errors; a new method of *diagnosis*; a correction of the fundamental errors of *metabolism*, high protein foods, blood circulation, blood composition, and last but not least, you must be taught:

What Vitality Really Is

To medical science, the human body is still a mystery, especially in a diseased condition.[8] Every new disease "discovered" by doctors is a new mystery for them. There are no words to express how far they are away from the truth. Naturopathy uses the word Vitality continually. Yet neither "medical scientists" nor naturopaths can tell what *Vitality* is.

Not only is it necessary to eradicate all these errors from your brain, but to show you the truth in such a new and simple light that you can grasp it at once. This great advantage of simplicity and clarity is one of the fundamental reasons for my success. Withal, my teachings cover the truth. Incidentally, *whatever simple reason* cannot be grasped is *humbug*, however *scientific* it may sound.

You will learn how wrong and ignorant it is to believe that any special disease can be healed by eating the right food, living on "special menus," or undergoing long fasts, if such is done without experience and without system, and special advice for each individual case.[9]

"Fasting" has been known for hundreds of years as "compensation" against every disease, as nature's only and infallible law, and the same with the mucusless diet, as already stated in Genesis (fruits and herbs, i.e., green leaves).[10] But why did it never

10

come into general use and resultant universal success? This is because it was never used systematically in accordance with the condition of the patient. The average man or woman has not the slightest idea what the necessary eliminative process is; what time it requires; how and how often their diet must be changed; or what it means to cleanse the body of the terrible quantities of waste that they have accumulated in their bodies during their lives.

Disease is an effort of the body to eliminate waste, mucus, and toxemias, and this system assists nature in the most perfect and natural way. Not the disease but the body is to be healed; it must be cleansed, freed from waste and foreign matter, from mucus and toxemias accumulated since childhood. You cannot buy health in a bottle, you cannot heal your body, that is, cleanse your system in a few days. You must make "compensation" for the wrong you have done your body all during your life.

My system is not a cure or a remedy, it is a regeneration, a thorough housecleaning, an acquisition of such clean and perfect health as you never knew before.

Remember: Your constitutional encumbrances throughout the entire system are the source of every disease; the greatest and most harmful source of lowered vitality, imperfect health, lack of strength and endurance, and any and all imperfect conditions. All disease has its source in the colon, never perfectly emptied since your birth. Nobody on earth today has an ideally clean body, and therefore perfectly clean blood. What medical science calls "normal health" is in fact a pathological condition.

In Summa: the human mechanism is an elastic pipe system. The diet of civilization is never entirely digested nor the resultant waste eliminated. This entire pipe system is slowly constipated, especially at the place of the symptom and the digestive tract. This is the foundation of every disease. To loosen this waste, eliminate it intelligently and carefully, and to control this operation can only be done perfectly, by the

MUCUSLESS DIET HEALING SYSTEM

[1] Many people assume that Ehret is referring only to bowel constipation. However, his use of the word is much broader in scope, referring to constitutional encumbrances on the cellular level that have been obstructing one's organism since birth. Although Ehret does assert that the foundation of cellular constipation is bowel constipation, which is the definite result of eating pus- and mucus-forming foods, Ehret's concept of the term extends beyond the bowels

[2] The word "mucus" is from the Latin *mucus* which means "slime, mold, snot, etc." Mucus refers to a thick, viscous, slippery discharge that is comprised of dead cells, mucin, inorganic salts, water, and exfoliated cells. It also refers to the slimy, sticky, viscous substance left behind by mucus-forming foods in the body after ingestion.

[3] This fact may be hard to believe at first. Later in this book, Ehret will discuss cases where he helped people eliminate a lot more than 10 pounds of fecal matter from the bowels. Also, since the time of Ehret, other naturopaths have observed and documented the elimination of pounds of mucoid plaque (rubber-like strings of rotting mucus found in the intestines), feces, decades-old feces stones, and other toxemias. To look at some compelling pictorial examples of such waste, see Bernard Jensen's *Tissue Cleansing through Bowel Management*. Keep in mind that most of the dietary prescriptions in the book are problematic, and I do not recommend using them. However, the real pictures of the kind of internal waste that humans harbor are profound.

[4] "Mucusless" refers to foods that are not mucus-forming. Such foods digest without leaving behind a thick, viscous, slimy substance called mucus. These foods include all kinds of fat-free and starchless fruits and vegetables.

[5] The word "fruit" refers to the ripened ovary or ovaries of a seed-bearing plant, together with accessory parts containing the seeds and occurring in a wide variety of forms. Ehret is specifically referring to mucusless fruits: fat-free and starchless fruits that leave behind no mucus residue. An unripe banana is an example of a starchy fruit, while an avocado is a fatty one. "Green leafy vegetables" refers to various mucusless leafy plants or their leaves and stems that may be eaten as vegetables.

[6] The word "fast" means to abstain from the intake of food and drink for a period of time. It may also refer to various forms of dietary restriction,

which include abstaining from solid foods (juice or liquid fasting), mucus-forming foods (mucusless diet), animal products, and so forth. Fasting may also refer more broadly to abstaining from modern conveniences or unnatural additions, for example, a fast from electricity or the use of electronics for a period of time.

"Mucus-forming" refers to foods that create or leave behind uneliminated mucus in the human body. Such foods include meats, dairy, grains, starches, and fats.

Ehret periodically uses the term "disease" to refer to human illness. Yet, Ehret suggests that the word is inherently problematic, hence appearing in quotations. With that said, Ehret does not ever purport to "treat" diseases, but to naturally heal human illness through a change in diet toward mucusless foods and short-term fasting. Since the initial publication of the *Mucusless Diet*, the use of the word "disease" by non-medical professionals has been vigorously contested. In many countries, people face legal consequences for diagnosing, or claiming to cure, what the medical profession refers to as "disease."

To gain insight into the meaning of the word disease, we must consider its etymology (historical origins). The term "disease" can be traced back to the early fourteenth century, when it meant "discomfort" or "inconvenience." It derives from the Old French "desaise" meaning "lack, want; discomfort, distress, trouble, misfortune, or sickness." Literally 'des (dis)' meaning "without, away" and "aise" or ease meaning comfort, pleasure, or well-being. The word was still commonly used in its literal sense until the early part of the seventeenth century, and has been revived in modern usage with the spelling *dis-ease*.

By the seventeenth century, the word "disease" was also being used to identify specific conditions of the body, or of some body part or organ, in which its functions are disturbed or deranged. Over time the word came to be used to identify a species of disorder or ailment, in which they exhibit special symptoms or affect a specific organ. Customarily the defining words of the "disease" either indicate its symptomatic nature, were derived from the surname of a person who has suffered from it, or the surname of the physician who first diagnosed it. For instance "Bright's Disease," the disease

13

Ehret was diagnosed with, and which he cured himself of, was first described in 1827 by the English physician Richard Bright.

Ehret tends to use the term "disease" in its original sense, which is to refer to a distressing or uncomfortable condition of the body. Yet, he identifies the express purpose of this condition to be "an effort of the body to eliminate waste, mucus, and toxemias." This is a significant definition of disease because it is one of the foundational concepts for the mucusless diet—that we eat for the purpose of cleansing and not to obtain nutritional sustenance. Yet, in subsequent lessons, Ehret does critique the medical notion of diseases, and shows how a mucusless diet expert can interpret and use medical diagnoses to determine what type of transition diet and fasting protocols to suggest to their patients.

[7] The term naturopathy was coined in 1895 by John Scheel and made famous in the United States by one of Ehret's students named Benedict Lust, who founded the first school of naturopathy in 1902. Naturopathic medicine favors a holistic and drugless approach to healing and seeks to find the least invasive measures necessary to relieve symptoms and heal human illness. "Natural Hygiene," or orthopathy, is a healing philosophy derived from naturopathy that advocates plant-based diets and periods of intermittent fasting. Although many prominent naturopaths and natural hygienic practitioners were, and continue to be, greatly influenced by Ehret's works, their healing practices and philosophies about nutrition usually greatly differ from Ehret's.

[8] "Science" comes from Latin "scientia," meaning "knowledge." The term refers to a systematic enterprise that builds and organizes knowledge in the form of testable explanations and predictions about the universe. Also, it may be identified to be the methodical study of the structure and behavior of the physical and natural world through observation and experimentation. "Medical science" refers to an institution specializing in the treatment of diseases.

[9] The term "system" in this sense refers to a set of principles or procedures according to which something is done, and/or an organized scheme or method. It is important to remember that the mucusless diet is a systematic approach to eating. It is important to not become overzealous and rush through or skip over aspects of the systematic transition discussed throughout the book.

[10] In Genesis 1:29, the voice of God tells Adam and Eve that their diet should consist of fruit. Although there are many different translations of the verse, they all have a similar meaning that suggests the first humans were at best fruitarians, or, at worst, raw, and mucusless fruit and vegetable eaters. One common variation is from the Vulgate, which is a late fourth-century Latin translation of the Bible: "*And God said, Behold, I have given you every herb [plant] bearing seed, which is upon the face of all the earth, and every tree, in which is the fruit of a tree yielding seed: to you it shall be for food* [meat]" (Vulgate translation).

According to this verse, the fruit of a tree yielding seed, as well as the seeded fruit from herbs (plants such as a grapevine), are to be the food of humans. Such foods perfectly situate humans into the circle of plant and animal life on this planet. In theory, when humans living in nature eat fruit, they either consume its seeds or discard them onto the fertile ground. Seeds that were eaten would eventually return to the earth following a bowel movement. The seeds then have the potential to germinate and produce a new tree or plant which will grow more fruit. Humans cannot eat processed foods or dead animal flesh and hope to directly produce more packaged foods or living animals.

Genesis 1:29 is the second utterance from God to humans. The first is in Genesis 1:28: "*And God blessed them, and God said unto them, Be fruitful, and multiply, and replenish the earth, and subdue it: and have dominion over the fish of the sea, and over the fowl of the air, and over every living thing that moveth upon the earth*" (Vulgate translation).

It must be pointed out that humans were to have dominion over animals, but not to eat them. In
fact, animals did not even have the right to eat other animals in Eden. Genesis 1:30 states: "*And to every beast of the earth, and to every fowl of the air, and to everything that creepeth upon the earth, wherein there is life, I have given every green herb for meat [food]: and it was so*" (Vulgate translation).

This would suggest that the first animals were inherently herbivores when not fully fruitarian. I point this out because many readers have interpreted "herbs" in Genesis 1:29 to signify that humans are also inherently vegetable eaters. My interpretation is that humans are to have the fruit from the herbs (plants). Thus, a grapevine is an herb that produces seed-bearing fruit. We need not eat the vine or its leaves, but the grapes that are produced from it.

With that said, Genesis 1:29 and 1:30 together offer the proposition of a mucus-free world inhabited by mucusless humans and animals.

In sum, volumes can and have been written about these several verses and principles of life on earth. Many spiritual and religious philosophies have suggested that superior humans are fruit eaters and frequent fasters. Christianity, Judaism, Jainism, Buddhism, Hinduism, Taoism, Islam, Ancient Egyptian Mystery Schools, and more all have strong fasting traditions, and many propagate various forms or degrees of fruit dieting. Ehret, a student of world culture and religion, took note of this fact and would periodically invoke Genesis 1:29 and discuss various fasting traditions in his teachings.

Latent, Acute, and Chronic Diseases—

No Longer a Mystery

Lesson II

The first lesson has now given you an insight as to what disease actually is. In addition to mucus and its toxemias in the system, there are other foreign matters such as uric acid, toxins, etc., and especially drugs, if ever used. I learned through years of practical experience that drugs are NEVER eliminated as is the waste from foods, but are stored up in the body for decades! Hundreds of cases have come under my observation where drugs taken 10, 20, 30, and even 40 years ago were expelled together with mucus through this perfect healing system. *This is a fact of basic importance—especially for the practitioner.* When these chemical poisons, after being dissolved, are taken back into circulation for elimination through the kidneys—the nerves and heart are affected—causing extreme nervousness, dizziness, and excessive heartbeats, as well as other strange sensations.[11] The uninformed stands before a mystery and probably calls the family doctor, who now diagnoses the condition as "heart disease" and blames the "lack of food" instead of the drugs he prescribed 10 years ago.

The average "normal" man or woman, considered healthy, has a chronic, stored-up accumulation of waste food, poisons, and drugs.

THIS IS HIS OR HER LATENT DISEASE

When these latent disease matters are occasionally stirred up, for instance by a cold, a person expels great quantities of mucus, and feels unhappy instead of enjoying nature's cleansing process. If the quantity of loosened mucus is great enough to more or less shock the entire system, but still not dangerous, it may be diagnosed as influenza. If the eliminating work of nature digs deeper into the system, especially into that important organ—the lungs—so much mucus and poisons are loosened at once that the circulation has to work under great friction, similar to a dirty machine—or, for example, an automobile running with its brakes set. The friction produces abnormal heat, which is called fever; the doctors call it pneumonia, which is really a "feverish" effort on nature's part to free the MOST VITAL organs from its waste. If the kidneys are called upon to eliminate this loosened mucus, thereby shocking this organ, it is called nephritis. In other words, whenever nature endeavors to save a human life through her efforts to "feverishly" eliminate mucus and its toxic products, it is called:

ACUTE DISEASE

The medical profession has over 4,000 names for different ailments.[12] The particular or special name of the disease is made up according to the respective local place of elimination; or to the congested point where the bloodstream finds a difficult passage and causes pain—such as pains in the joints, as in cases of rheumatism.

For ages, this well-meaning effort and intended self-healing work of nature has been misunderstood and suppressed through the agency of drugs and the continuance of eating, despite the warning danger signals of pain and loss of appetite. Notwithstanding the "help" of the doctors—a help, in fact, injurious and dangerous to the patient's life—their vitality and especially their eliminating abilities are lowered, and nature proceeds slowly. Under this handicap, nature cannot work as efficiently, requiring more time, and the case is called "chronic." The word chronic is derived from the Greek word "chronos," meaning time. You will be taught more about this mystery in Lessons 3 and 4.

[11] The word "elimination" refers to the removal of physiological wastes and encumbrances from the bloodstream, lymph system, or body. The term is also used by many practitioners of the *Mucusless Diet Healing System* to identify short or extended periods of intensive waste elimination. These practitioners use the term instead of the word *sick*, as the connotation of the latter is believed to be problematic. In parlance, a practitioner may say "I'm going through an intense elimination today!" meaning that he or she is presumably eliminating large quantities of waste and experiencing various symptoms of human illness. Instances of elimination usually spur a practitioner to detoxify, fast, or abstain from mucus-forming foods. As waste is loosened, the body will try to eliminate it by any means necessary. Elimination may occur through the bowels, kidneys, skin, sinuses, eyes, ears, hair, mouth, and so forth.

[12] In 2007, the World Health Organization distinguished over 12,420 disease categories. This number increases every year.

Why the Diagnosis

Lesson III

Why The Diagnosis?

Laymen and even some dietetic experts, with exception of myself, believe there is no need for diagnosis.[13] You may ask, since there is only one disease, why the diagnosis? If all sickness is due to uncleanliness caused by uneliminated, undigested food, mucus, uric acid, toxemias, drugs, and so forth, why diagnose? We shall now learn why fruit diet and fasting have produced such doubtful results through their incorrect use and misunderstanding, caused by the belief that general rules of this cure are suitable for everybody and for every case. Nothing is further from the truth! No other cure requires so much individual specialization and continual changing to meet the reaction of the patient. This is why people who attempt these methods of cure without expert advice frequently bring about serious results.

Promiscuous Fasting

Macfadden[14] and many others, for instance, advised fasting as applicable to all cases. I learned through thousands of cases during my experience that nothing requires more individual, different application than fasting and the mucusless diet. Of two patients, one may recover completely after a fast of 2 or 3 weeks, while the other may die from the same treatment! That is why an individual diagnosis of general conditions and constitutional encumbrances is so necessary.

Method of Constitutional Diagnosis

My diagnosis determines the following points:

1. The relative amount of encumbrance in the system,

2. The predominant part, that is, whether more mucus or more poisons,

3. If pus is present in the system, and the amount and kind of drugs used,[15]

4. If internal tissue or an organ is in a process of decomposition, and

5. How far vitality is lowered.

You will also learn through experience and observations along these lines that the general appearance, especially the face of the patient, will indicate more or less the internal condition.

Medical Diagnosis

Medical diagnosis throws no real light on the subject, although doctors think it more important than the actual cure. It is made up of a series of reports of symptoms and a scheme of experiences from which thousands of diseases are named. Characteristic of the meaningless medical diagnosis is the frequent statement of many patients that "the doctors could not find out what I have." THE NAME OF THE DISEASE DOES NOT CONCERN US AT ALL. A person with gout, one with indigestion, or one with Bright's disease may start with the same advice. Whether to fast, for instance, and how long, does not depend upon the name of the disease, but upon the patient's condition and how far vitality is lowered.

Naturopathic Concepts

Naturopathy is an advance over medicine in teaching that all disease is constitutional. Yet, naturopathy does not explain sufficiently the source, nature, and composition of "foreign matters" as the fundamental one-ness of all disease.

Dr. Lahmann[16] said: "Every disease is caused by carbonic acid and gas." But he did not learn its source in decayed, uneliminated food substance: the mucus in a state of continuous fermentation.

Dr. Jaeger[17] said, "Disease is a stench." Nature gives a diagnosis through bad odor, which indicates how far the inside decomposition has progressed.

Dr. Haig[18] of England, the founder of the "Anti-uric-acid Diet," based his conception of general diagnosis on the assumption that the majority of diseases are caused through uric acid, certainly an important part of diseased matter besides mucus.

Naturopathy puts considerable stress and importance on symptomatic diagnosis in spite of the acknowledgment that there is only one disease.

Uric Diagnosis

Medical doctors and many others consider this special kind of diagnosis as the most important one, but it is fundamentally misunderstood. Besides the digestive tract, the uric canal is the main avenue of elimination. *As soon as any one decreases their eating, fasts a little, or changes over to the natural diet, he or she has waste, mucus, poisons, uric acid, phosphates, and so on,* in their urine, and an analysis of this urine is alarming. The same thing happens in the majority of cases whenever anyone becomes sick. Every one becomes alarmed at this effort of the body to eliminate waste—which is, in truth, the healing, cleansing process.

Should sugar or albumen be found in the urine, the case is called "very serious," and diagnosed as "Diabetes" or "Bright's disease," respectively. Under medical treatment, the patient in the first named case dies through sugar-starvation, caused through lack of sugar and sugar-formers in the diet.[19] In the latter diagnosis, the patient dies from forced "albumen replacement," resulting from overfeeding of foods rich in albumen.[20]

WHATEVER THE BODY EXPELS IS WASTE, DECAYED, DEAD—and simply indicates that the patient is in an advanced state of inside uncleanliness, already causing a decomposition of inside organs—producing rapid decay of all food taken into the body.

These cases, like tuberculosis, must be treated *very carefully* and *VERY SLOWLY*.

How It Looks in the Human Colon

It is of utmost importance that through our diagnoses we must learn as much as possible the general appearance of the inside of the human body. Our diagnosis therefore consists in finding out the degree of quantities of individual waste matter of the patient.

Experts in autopsy state they have found that from 60 percent to 70 percent of the colons examined have foreign matters such as worms and decades-old feces-stones. The inside walls of the over-intestines are encrusted by old, hardened feces and resemble in appearance the inside of a filthy stovepipe.

I had obese patients that eliminated from their body as much as 50 to 60 pounds of waste, and 10 to 15 pounds alone from the colon—mainly consisting of foreign matters, especially old, hardened, feces. The average so-called "healthy" person of today carries continually with them, since childhood, several pounds of never-eliminated feces. One "good stool" a day means nothing. A fat and sick person is in fact a living "cesspool." A distinct surprise to me was that a number of my patients in such condition had already undertaken so-called "nature cures."

---

[13] Neither Ehret nor the editor of this book purports to "diagnose" medical diseases. Ehret uses the word diagnosis to simply mean the interpretation of health issues based upon observable physiological factors. Ehret's approach may be identified as the *Mucusless Diet Healing System* diagnosis, as it is different from medical, and even many naturopathic, diagnostic approaches. As mentioned in Lesson II, the medical name of a disease is not particularly important, although such information may be used to determine the best way to apply the *Mucusless Diet Healing System*.

[14] Bernarr Macfadden (1868–1955) was an influential American proponent of physical culture and health. He also founded the long-running magazine publishing company, Macfadden Publications. One of his most famous magazines, *Physical Culture*, was first published in 1899. He was the

predecessor of Charles Atlas and Jack LaLanne, and has been credited with helping to begin the culture of health and fitness in the United States. Macfadden was a strong proponent of fasting and felt that it was the best way to achieve physical health. Many of his subjects would fast for a week with the goal of rejuvenating their body. He claimed that "a person could exercise unqualified control over virtually all types of disease while revealing a degree of strength and stamina such as would put others to shame" through fasting.

[15] The word "pus" is from late fourteenth-century Latin "pus" (related to puter [putrid] "rotten"), from Proto-Indo-European *pu- compared to Sanskrit puyati "rots, stinks," putih "stinking, foul." Pus often refers to a thick white, yellowish, or greenish opaque liquid produced in infected tissue, consisting of dead white blood cells, bacteria, tissue debris, and serum. It also refers to the substance that dead animal flesh is chemically changed to after being consumed or while rotting. Thus, the ingestion of meat and dairy products create pus residue in the body.

[16] Johann Heinrich Lahmann (1860-1905) was a German physician and pioneer of naturopathic medicine. He earned his medical doctorate at the University of Heidelberg, and became a general practitioner in Stuttgart. On 1 January 1888, he opened a sanatorium called the "Physiatric Sanatorium" at Weißer Hirsch, outside of Dresden, which became internationally known. He eventually abandoned traditional medicine as he became disdainful of drugs and unnatural medications. He became a proponent of a vegetarian diet, exercise, and fresh air, and was an ardent practitioner of physiotherapy and hydrotherapy.

[17] Gustav Jaeger (1832-1917) was a German naturalist, hygienist, and professor of zoology. In 1884, he abandoned teaching and started practice as a physician in Stuttgart. He advanced the first version of the pheromone concept and wrote various works on biological subjects. He also advocated wearing rough animal-based fabrics, such as wool, in close proximity to the skin and objected to the use of plant fibers like cotton. His teachings inspired the creation of the Jaeger clothing brand (1884).

[18] Alexander Haig, MD (1853-1924) was the author of several books on diet and human illness. He is known for his theory that "uric acid" and foods that promote uric acid in the body are the foundation of human illness. For further reading, see *Uric Acid: An Epitome of the Subject* (1906) and *Uric acid as a factor in the causation of disease; a contribution to the pathology of high blood pressure,*

25

headache, epilepsy, nervousness, mental disease, asthma, hay fever, paroxysmal hæmoglobinuria, anæmia, Bright's disease, diabetes, gout, rheumatism, bronchitis, and other disorders (1908).

[19] Ehret is referring to the handful of illnesses in which medical doctors order people to avoid eating fruit and tell them to eat albuminous, or pus-forming, foods. From Ehret's perspective, this is very problematic, as he finds mucusless fruits to be the key to cleaning the body and healing it. In such cases where fruit produces uncomfortable and dangerous symptoms, Ehret suggests that the patient must control their eliminations by eating a more vegetable-heavy transition diet integrated with short periods of fasting (this will be covered in subsequent lessons).

It must also be noted that simple sugars (carbohydrates), particularly fructose, which Ehret often refers to as grape or fruit sugar, is instrumental to healing. Simple sugars (monosaccharides) should never be confused with complex sugars (or complex carbohydrates) that come from starch, milk, etc., which are injurious to the body and should be avoided.

[20] The word "albumen," also spelled "albumin," was originally used to refer to the "white of an egg," deriving from Latin albumen, literally "whiteness," from albus "white." It is a class of simple, water-soluble proteins that can be coagulated by heat and are found in egg whites, blood serum, milk, and many other animal and plant tissues. Albuminous refers to something consisting of, resembling, or containing albumen. Albuminous foods decompose into pus inside the body.

The Diagnosis—Part 2

Lesson IV

Fat and Lean Types

The bodily mechanism of the fat type is, on the average, *mechanically* more obstructed because he or she is, in general, an overeater of starchy foods. In the lean type, there is more *physiological* chemical interference with the organism, such as one being in general a one-sided meat eater, a condition which produces especially much acidity, uric acid, other poisons, and pus.[21]

Disease Story

As a general rule, I ask my prospective patients the following questions, as the knowledge to be gained is of great importance:

1. How long have you been sick?

2. What did the doctor call your disease?

3. What was the nature of the treatment?

4. How much and what kinds of treatment was taken?

5. Have you ever been operated on?

6. What other kinds of treatment have you taken before?

(Age, sex, whether a disease is inherited, etc., are important points.)

The most important thing, however, is the patient's diet at present, their special craving for certain foods, their wrong habits, and if constipated, and how long. What kinds of diets, if any, were used before? It is necessary to base the change in diet on the patient's present diet, and only a SLIGHT CHANGE toward an improved diet is advisable.[22]

The Experimental Diagnosis

THE MOST EXACT, UNERRING DIAGNOSIS WE HAVE IS A SHORT FAST. The more rapidly the patient feels "worse" through a short fast, the greater and the more poisonous is his or her encumbrance. Should they become dizzy, suffer severe headaches, etc.; they are greatly clogged up with mucus and toxemias. If palpitation of the heart occurs, *it is a sign that pus is somewhere in the system*, or that drugs, even though taken many years ago, are in the circulation for elimination.

Any inside special "constipated" place is located by a light pain there. The experimental practitioner can ascertain better than with X-rays, through nature's revelation after a short fast, the true condition of the inside of the human body, and knows the real diagnosis more correctly than doctors can ascertain with all their expensive scientific equipment and instruments.

If this "short-fast" diagnosis is tried on the average person called normal and healthy—but in reality clogged up with mucus and latent disease—nature reveals the same in a moderate degree. If a "weak point" has begun to develop, unsuspected by them, nature will unerringly indicate where and how he or she will later become sick if the wrong method of living is continued, although it may be after some years. This then, is the PROGNOSIS OF DISEASE.

Some Special Diagnoses

To show that all differently named diseases, even the most severe ones, have their basis and are caused by the same general and constitutional encumbrance of the body, I shall show you, in the light of truth, a few characteristic kinds of cases. Through these *illustrative examples*, I shall prove that there is not a single disease, not a

28

disturbance or sensation, not an unhealthy appearance or symptom, which cannot be explained and seen at once in its real nature as local constipation, constitutional constipation, by mucus and its toxemias; most of the quantities continually supplied from the "chronic reserve stock of waste" in the stomach, intestines, and especially, in the colon. The "basement" of the human "temple" is the reservoir from which every symptom of disease and weakness is supplied in all its manifestations.

A COLD

It is a beneficial effort to eliminate waste from the cavities of the head, the throat, and the bronchial tubes.

PNEUMONIA

The cold goes deeper and will eliminate and clean the mucus from the most spongy and vital organ, the lung. A hemorrhage occurs to clean more radically. The entire system is aroused, causing higher temperature by friction of the waste in circulation. That proves alarming, and the doctor suppresses this by drugs and food, and thus actually blocks nature's process of healing—cleansing. If the patient does not die, the elimination becomes chronic and is called

CONSUMPTION[23]

The consumptive patient continually eliminates his or her mucus caused from erroneously increased, mucus-forming foods through the lungs instead of through natural ways. This organ itself decays more and more, producing germs; and it is then called tuberculosis.

The vital organ (lung)—the pump—works insufficiently on the circulation, the entire cell system decays more and more, and decomposes before the patient dies.

TOOTHACHE

Its pain is a warning signal of nature: "Stop eating; I must repair; there is waste and pus; you have eaten too much lime-poor food, meat."[24]

RHEUMATISM AND GOUT

Mucus and uric acid particularly accumulate in the joints, since there is the less dependable part of the tissues for the passage of the circulation, heavily loaded with waste and uric acid in the one-sided meat eater's body.

STOMACH TROUBLE

The stomach is the central organ of disease matter supply. There is a limit to the ability of this organ to digest and to empty itself after the meal. Every type of food (even the best kinds) is mixed with this acid mucus, continually remaining in the average person's stomach. The wonder is how long the human being can stand such conditions.[25]

GOITER

It is a deposit, by nature, of tremendous waste to keep it from entering the circulation.

A BOIL

It is in principle the same as a goiter, only the elimination is outside.

STAMMERING

It is a special accumulation of mucus in the throat, interfering with the functioning of the vocal chords. I have cured several cases.[26]

LIVER AND KIDNEY DISEASES

These organs are of a very spongy construction, and their function is that of a kind of physiological sieve. They are, therefore, easily constipated by sticky mucus.[27]

SEX DISEASES

These have for their origin nothing more than mucus elimination through these organs, and are easily healed. The use of drugs alone produces the characteristic symptoms of syphilis. The more drugs that have been used, especially mercury, the more carefully the treatment must be conducted.[28]

EAR AND EYE DISEASES

Even short- or far-sightedness is congestion in the eyes, and trouble with hearing from congestion of those organs. I healed a few kinds of blindness and deafness by the same principles.[29]

MENTAL DISEASES

Besides a congested system, I found that anyone mentally diseased has congestion, especially of the brain. One man on the verge of insanity was cured by a 4-week fast. There is nothing easier to heal by fasting than insanity—such men and women, having lost their reason, their natural instinct tells them not to eat. I learned that if you heal through the *Mucusless Diet Healing System* all kinds of illnesses, most of the patients are relieved of greater or lesser mental conditions. After a fast comes a clearer mind. Unity of ideas comes to take the place of differences. Differences of ideas today are caused largely by diet. If something is wrong with anyone, look first to the stomach. The mentally diseased man or woman suffers physiologically from gas pressure on the brain.

---

[21] Arnold Ehret categorizes human physiology into two main categories: fat (also called mucus) and lean (also called uric acid) types. People with uric acid physiologies are often said to have "high metabolisms," and can seemingly eat a lot and not gain any weight. The misconception is that this person is healthier than an overweight person. This is often not the case, as their body only handles mucus and pus differently than someone with a fatty or mucus physiology. This condition often occurs in people who are one-sided meat eaters, a condition that produces uric acid, other poisons, and pus. Essentially, instead of depositing mucus as fat throughout the organism, such waste is converted to poisonous acid. Low-carb diets that emphasize eating meat, such as the Atkins Diet, essentially transform one's body type from fat to lean. Thus, weight loss for people on such a diet is a negative proposition because they lose weight at the expense of creating much internal toxicity. Thin people who participate in competitive eating are usually lean, uric acid types. Contrarily, when someone with a fat, mucus type of physiology eats pus- and mucus-forming foods, it will usually result in weight gain. Eating great amounts of such foods is the cause of obesity in people with this type of physiology.

²² One of the most misunderstood and often ignored elements of the *Mucusless Diet Healing System* is the recommendation to adhere to "only a SLIGHT CHANGE toward an improved diet" at first. Although this is discussed in detail throughout the book, many people who endeavor to practice the diet without expert assistance try to skip the transition and go directly into long fasts and aggressive fruit diets. It cannot be emphasized enough how wrong such an approach is. Ehret does not recommend any patient do long fasts or extended fruit dieting in the beginning. What does a "slight change" in diet look like? What is too slight and what is too aggressive? These questions will be explored further in subsequent lessons.

²³ "Consumption" is an archaic term for what is currently referred to as pulmonary tuberculosis. Ehret's discussion may also be generally applied to all "obstructive lung diseases," which are respiratory illness characterized by airway obstruction. Terms used to denote various forms of constipation of the lungs include asthma, bronchiectasis, bronchitis, and chronic obstructive pulmonary disease (COPD).

²⁴ By "lime-poor," Ehret is referring to foods that lack minerals. Consider the concept of "lime-rich" soil which is highly alkaline and may be used to neutralize acidity. From Ehret's perspective, the importance of mineral-rich foods is their cleansing properties.

²⁵ For a detailed exploration of the fetid internal condition of the human stomach, see Ehret's book, *Thus Speaketh the Stomach*. In this unique work, Ehret gives voice to the stomach through a first-person perspective that allows the reader to intimately explore the foundation of human illness.

²⁶ Today, "stammering" is more commonly referred to as "stuttering" or "disfluency." It is a type of communication and speech issue where a person speaks with sudden involuntary pauses and a tendency to repeat the initial letters of words.

²⁷ Most people, no matter how healthy they seem, have weakened kidneys. As a result, they fail to filter as much cellular waste from their body as they should. As you progress with the mucusless diet, your urine may become very yellow or contain sediment. This happens as the kidneys begin to better filter the accumulated wastes that you are now loosening.

²⁸ Mercury is no longer used to treat venereal diseases. As early as the 1300s, it was used as a treatment for skin conditions, and there are reports

of it being used to treat syphilis in 1496. Mercury is toxic to humans, and although the treatment harmed many people, it was commonly used for over three centuries. During the early 1900s, non-mercury treatments for venereal diseases developed, and scientific studies on mercury poisoning, notably from the German chemist Alfred Stock, confirmed to other members of the scientific community its toxicity to humans. Although its use for venereal diseases fell out of fashion, mercury-based dental amalgam fillings continue to the present day in the midst of much controversy. If you had, or have, mercury fillings, you will want to be careful as you begin to use the *Mucusless Diet Healing System*. When the dormant poisons from heavy metals begin to reenter your system in order to be eliminated, many unpleasant symptoms may arise. In general, be careful to not be too aggressive with strict fasts or fruit-only periods while you are eliminating these poisons. For support and guidance in safely confronting mercury-related issues using the mucusless diet, it is advisable to seek assistance from an expert *Mucusless Diet Healing System* practitioner.

[29] In addition to congestion, eye strain can also cause eye issues. To learn about methods that have helped people remove eye strain, see William Horatio Bates' (1860–1931) *Perfect Sight without Glasses* (1920). Support groups with modern practitioners of the *Bates Method* are also accessible online.

The Magic Mirror

Lesson IVa

Supplement to Diagnosis

Since humans degenerated through civilization, they no longer know what to do when they become sick. Disease remains the same mystery to modern medical science as it was to the "medicine man" of thousands of years ago—the main difference being that the "germ" theory has replaced the "demon" and that mysterious, outside power remains—to harm you and destroy your life.

Disease is a mystery to you as well as to every doctor who has not as yet looked into the "magic mirror" which I am about to explain. Naturopathy deserves full credit for having proven that disease is within you—a foreign matter which has weight—and which must be eliminated.

If you want to become your own physicians, or, if you are a drugless healer and if you want more success, you must learn the truth and know what diseases are. You cannot heal yourself or other people without an exact diagnosis which will give you a clear idea of true conditions. This infallible truth can be learned only from the book of Nature: that is, through a test on your own body—or the "magic mirror," as I have designated it.

35

The sufferer from any kind of disease—or any person, whether sick or not—who will go through the healing process of fasting and mucusless diet, will eliminate mucus—thereby demonstrating that the basic cause of all latent diseases of humans are a clogged-up tissue system of uneliminated, unused and undigested food substances.

Through the "magic mirror" a true and unfailing diagnosis of your disease is furnished, as never before.

"THE MAGIC MIRROR"

1. Proof that your personal, individual symptom, sore, or sensation, according to what your disease is named, is nothing more than an extraordinary local accumulation of waste.

2. The coated tongue is evidence of a constitutional encumbrance throughout the entire system, which obstructs and congests the circulation by dissolved mucus, and this mucus even appears in the urine.

3. The presence of unevacuated feces, retained through sticky mucus in the pockets of the intestines, constantly poisoning, and thereby interfering with proper digestion and blood building.

To look inside your body—far better and clearer than can be done by doctors with expensive X-ray apparatus—and learn the cause of your disease, or even discover some hitherto unknown physical imperfection or mental condition, try this:

Fast 1 or 2 days, or eat fruits only (such as oranges, apples, or any juicy fruit in season) for 2 or 3 days, and you will notice that your tongue will become heavily coated. When this happens to the acutely sick, the doctor's conclusion is always "indigestion." The tongue is the mirror not only of the stomach, but of the entire membrane system as well. The fact that this heavy coating returns, even if removed by a tongue scraper once or twice a day, is an accurate indication of the amount of filth, mucus, and other poisons accumulated in the tissues of your entire system, now being eliminated on the inside surface of the stomach, intestines and every cavity of your body.

You will become further convinced of this fact—of this diagnosis of your disease—by another surprise in store for you; if you will empty your intestines both before and after the test.

During the fast you are truly on Nature's operating table without the use of a knife! The cleansing eliminating process begins immediately and the knowledge contained in these lessons provide the needed information necessary to secure the desired results.

After you have fasted, it is advisable to decrease the quantity of your customary amount of food—and eat only natural, cleansing, mucusless foods (fruits and starchless vegetables), thereby affording the body an opportunity to loosen and eliminate mucus, which is, in fact,

THE HEALING PROCESS.

This "mirror" on the tongue's surface reveals to the observer the amount of encumbrance that has been clogging up the system since childhood—through wrong, mucus-forming foods. After observing the urine during this test, by allowing it to stand for a few hours, you will note the elimination of quantities of mucus in the same.

The actual amount of filth and waste, which is the "mysterious" cause of your "trouble," is almost unbelievable.

Every disease is first a special, local constipation of the circulation, tissues, pipe system and hence the manifestation of symptoms, or, of the different symptoms. If painful and inflamed, it is from overpressure—heat or inflammation caused by friction and congestion.

Second: Disease—every disease— is constitutional constipation. The entire human pipe system, especially the microscopically small capillaries, is "chronically" constipated through the wrong food of civilization.

White blood corpuscles are waste—and there is no man or woman in Western civilization who has mucus-free blood and mucus-free blood vessels. It is like the soot in a stovepipe which has never been cleaned; in fact, worse—because the waste from protein and starchy foods is STICKY.

37

The characteristics of tissue construction, especially of the important internal organs, such as the lungs, kidneys, all glands, etc., are very much similar to those of a sponge. Imagine a sponge soaked in paste or glue!

Naturopathy must cleanse its science from medical superstitions—wrongly called "scientific diagnosis." Nature, alone, is the teacher of a standard science of truth. She heals through one thing—FASTING—every disease that it is possible to heal. This, alone, is proof that Nature recognizes but one disease and that in everybody the largest factors are always waste, foreign matter, and mucus (besides uric acid and other toxemias, and very often, pus—if tissues are decomposed).

In order to realize how terribly clogged up the human body is, one must have seen thousands of people who fast—as I have. The almost inconceivable fact is: How can such quantities of waste be stored up in the body? Have you ever stopped to realize that masses of phlegm you expel during a cold? And just as it is taking place in your head—your bronchial tubes, lungs, stomach, kidneys, bladder, etc., have the same appearance. All are in the same condition. And the spongy organ known as the tongue accurately mirrors on its surface the appearance of every other part of your body.

Medicine has devised a "special science" of laboratory tests, urinal diagnoses, and blood tests.

More than 50 years ago, the most prominent pioneers of Naturopathy said: "Every disease is foreign matter—waste." I said 20 years ago and repeat it again and again, that most of these foreign matters are paste produced from wrong foods, decomposed—to be seen when it leaves the body as mucus. Meat decomposes into pus.

The light of truth dawned upon me after I had fasted against the will of the Naturopath from whom I was taking treatments for Bright's disease. When the test tube filled up with albumen, I read his thoughts in his facial expression. But to me, it proved that whatever Nature expels—eliminates—is waste; whether it be albumen, sugar, mineral salts, or uric acid. This occurred more than 24 years ago, but this Nature doctor (a former MD) still believes in the replacement of albumen in high protein foods.

38

The medical diagnosis of Bright's disease, when the chemical test of urine shows a high percentage of albumen, is as misleading as the others are. The elimination of albumen proves that the body does not need it, that it is overfed—overloaded with high protein stuff. Instead of decreasing these poison-producing foods, they are wrongly increased—endeavoring to replace the "loss"—until the patient dies. How tragic to replace waste, while Nature is endeavoring to save you by removing it!

The next important laboratory test is that of sugar in the urine— diabetes. The medical dictionary still calls it "mysterious." Instead of eating natural sweets, which go into the blood, and which can be used—the diabetic patient is fed eggs, meat, bacon, etc., and, in fact, actually starves to death through lack of natural, sugar-containing and sugar-producing foods, which have been withheld.

It has long since been proven that all of these blood tests, especially the Wasserman test, are a fallacy.

We, as Naturopaths, cannot ignore Nature's teaching in any way, even though we may find it difficult to discard old errors hammered into us since childhood.[30]

One of the most misleading errors is the individual naming of all diseases. The name of any disease is not important and not of any value whatsoever when starting a natural cure—especially through fasting and diet. If every disease is caused through foreign matters— and it most assuredly is—then it is only important and necessary to know how great and how much the amount of the patient's encumbrance actually is—how far and how much their system is clogged up by foreign matters, how much their vitality has become lowered (see Lesson V), and in case of tuberculosis or cancer, if the tissues themselves are decomposed (pus and germs).

I have had hundreds of cases tell me that every doctor they called upon gave a different diagnosis, and correspondingly different name for their ailment. I always surprise them by saying: "I know exactly what ails you—through facial diagnosis—and you will see it yourself in the 'magic mirror' within a few days."

39

The Experimental Diagnosis

Just as I have already stated in the beginning of this lesson, you must fast for 2 or 3 days.[31] The surface of the tongue will clearly indicate the appearance on the inside of the body, and the patient's breath will prove the amount and grade of decomposition. It is even possible to tell the kind of food they preferred most!

Should pain be felt at any one place, during the beginning of the fast, you may be sure that this is a weak point—and the symptom is not sufficiently developed for medical doctors to reveal it through their examination.

Waste will show up in the urine with clouds of mucus, and mucus will be expelled from the nose, throat, and lungs as well as in the feces. The weaker and more miserable the patient may feel during the fast, the greater is his or her encumbrance, and the weaker his or her vitality.

This experimental diagnosis tells you exactly what the trouble is, and how to correct it by starting with a moderate transition diet—or a more radical one—and whether to continue or discontinue the fast.

This experiment is the foundation—the basis of the development of the science of Nature cure, physics, chemistry, etc. It is the question put to Nature, and she replies with the same infallible answer, always and everywhere.

If a patient becomes nervous, or symptoms of heart trouble occur, you may be sure that they have drugs stored up in their body. A consumptive patient starts with such terrible elimination after a short fast that it must be plain to all how ignorant and how impossible it is to try to cure him with "good nourishing foods" such as eggs and milk.

The above explanation is the experimental diagnosis, and the only scientific one. You cannot secure a better view inside than by this simple method. No expensive apparatus can show more accurately the exact conditions as they exist inside the body. All other examination, including iris-diagnosis, diagnosis of the spine, etc., are never exact, and therefore, not dependable.

Nature's mirrors, her revelations, her demonstrations, and her phenomena are "magic" only so long as you lack the correct interpretation of them. Nature shows and plainly reveals to you everything—far more exact, perfect, and better than all "science of diagnosis" put together.

The Prognosis of Disease

And now we come to the prognosis of disease. We hear of "latent" disease. Everyone, no matter to what extent they may enjoy "good health," has a latent sickness—and Nature only awaits an opportunity to eliminate the waste stored up since childhood and on.

Everyone knows, but fails to understand, that a severe "shock," such as a cold—or "influenza" over the entire body—starts an elimination, but unfortunately, Nature is handicapped in her attempted housecleaning through the doctor's advice to continue eating, through the use of drugs, etc., obstructing elimination and producing acute and chronic diseases.

Anyone, even though not sick—especially in the critical stage between 30- and 40-years old—may fast a few days, and through the "magic mirror," learn the extent of their latent disease and where their weak point is located—as well as the name of their latent disease and where it will appear. That is the prognosis of disease, and if life insurance companies would only believe in it, would furnish a true and safe method of determining "risks."

Fasting until the tongue is clean is dangerous.[32] Who can explain why the tongue becomes clean after breaking a short fast with a "square" meal and why the "magic mirror" shows more waste, if you live on fruits or mucusless diet, after the fast? This is the hitherto unexplained mystery of the "Magic Mirror." And the simple explanation is that the elimination is stopped for a while, through the eating of wrong foods—and as a result you feel better for a time with wrong foods than with fruits. And during this period, even the "Magic Mirror" apparently leads you into thinking the body is clean. A return to natural foods soon proves otherwise.[33]

For the ordinary person, it will require from 1 to 3 years of systematically continued fasting and natural, cleansing diet before the body is actually cleansed of "foreign matters."[34] You may then see

41

how the body is constantly eliminating waste through the entire outside surface of the body, from every pore of the skin, the urinal canal, and the colon, from the eyes and ears, and from the nose and throat. You can see how wet as well as dry mucus (dandruff, for instance), is being expelled. All diseases, therefore, are immense quantities of waste, "chronically" stored up, and through this artificial elimination of "chronic disease," you will agree with me, and realize that I am not exaggerating when I state:

The diagnosis of your disease—of all diseases of humankind, both mental and physical, since the beginning of civilization, proves that they all have the same foundational cause—whatever the symptoms may be. It is, without exception, one and the same general and universal condition—a one-ness of all disease, that is: waste, foreign matter, mucus, and its poisons.

"Internal impurity" is too mild an expression for chronic constipation. Waste—filth—mucus—stench (offensive odor) or "invisible waste" are the true descriptions.

---

[30] Earlier in the text, Ehret critiques naturopathy suggesting that it "does not explain sufficiently the source, nature, and composition of 'foreign matters' as the fundamental one-ness of all disease." (See Naturopathic Concepts.) Yet, Ehret does identify himself as naturopath. Essentially, he contributes a much needed perspective to the discipline. Ehret's methods may be viewed as "true naturopathy."

[31] In most cases, liquids should be used during the fast. For full instructions on how to fast safely and effectively, see Fasting Lessons Part 1 through 4.

[32] Not only is fasting until the tongue is free of mucus dangerous, but depending upon the quantity of your internal uncleanliness, it can be near impossible early in your transition.

[33] The "Magic Mirror" can be a very helpful and enlightening tool to understand and use. Yet, it is important to put it into its proper perspective and not obsess over it. As Ehret says, your goal should not be to try to fast all of the mucus off your tongue at once. It takes years, perhaps decades, to totally clean the body to the point where your tongue will not secrete excess

mucus. Yet, the "Magic Mirror" can remind us that our body is one whole organism and not merely a collection of unrelated parts. In Western society, we have been conditioned to think about the body as a bunch of individual parts. Bones, organs, vessels, etc., can become compartmentalized in our consciousness. Yet, the mucus that is secreted from your tongue is the same that is being secreted along the walls of your stomach, intestines, and colon. Your entire digestive tract may be viewed as one long, continuous tube that goes from your mouth to your colon.

Many people wonder why they end up with a mouthful of mucus after eating fruit. This causes some to erroneously believe that the fruit is causing the mucus. Now, you may understand that the astringent properties of the fruit are pulling on the mucus membrane and causing the release of excess mucus. If your body is encumbered with waste, then the release of mucus in this way is necessary; yet as you rid your body of mucus, this kind of elimination happens less and less.

[34] Many beginners of the mucusless diet wonder how long it will take to totally cleanse the body. Ehret says, "For the ordinary person, it will require from 1 to 3 years of systematically continued fasting and natural, cleansing diet before the body is actually cleansed of 'foreign matters'." However, this statement is often misinterpreted to mean that it will only take 1 to 3 years to reach the highest levels of a mucusless lifestyle. In actuality, transitioning for 1 to 3 years is only the beginning of the process. If you have followed the program, within the first several years you should have eliminated the pounds of excess fecal matter from your bowels and started to deeply cleanse on the cellular level. But, based on the experiences of many long-term practitioners of the mucusless diet, it takes decades to totally cleanse the body and reach the highest levels. Yet, this should not deter you, as I suggest that you not be concerned with "how long" the diet will take. Time is relative to each person and we did not produce our physical ailments overnight. We must make compensation for the past, and it will take time. The key is to keep transitioning!

The Formula of Life

Lesson V

The Secret of Vitality

$V = P - O$ (V equals P minus O) is the formula of life—and at the same time, you may call it the formula of death.

"V" stands for VITALITY.

"P" or call it "X," the unknown quantity in this question, is the POWER that drives the human machinery, which keeps you alive, which gives you strength and efficiency—endurance for as yet an unknown length of time without food!

"O" means OBSTRUCTION, encumbrance, foreign matter, toxemias, mucus—in short, all internal impurities which obstruct the circulation, the function of internal organs especially, and the human engine in its entire functioning system.

You can therefore see through this equation that as soon as "O" becomes greater than "P" the human machine must come to a standstill.

The engineer can figure exactly "$E = P - F$," meaning that the amount of energy or efficiency "E" he or she secures from an engine is not equal to the power "P" without first deducting "F," the friction.

45

The ingenious idea of construction of the ideal engine is to make it work with the smallest amount of friction. Should we transfer this fundamental and principal idea to the human engine, we see that it involves the terrible ignorance of medical physiology, and that naturopathy found a true way of healing by removing or eliminating obstructions—that is, foreign matters of encumbrance, mucus, and its toxemias.

But just what vitality really is and how tremendous it can become; what a higher, superior absolute health is—has not up to the present date been shown or proven. I will teach in the following lessons a principally different NEW PHYSIOLOGY, based on the correction of medical errors of blood-circulation, blood-composition, blood-building, and metabolism. For this purpose, it is necessary that you first learn what vitality—what animal life—really is.

It is generally admitted that the secret of vitality, the secret of animal life, is unknown to science. It will surprise you when shown the truth through a simple, natural enlightenment, and you must admit at once that it is THE TRUTH. Always remember this fact: "Whatever cannot be seen—conceived at once—through simple reasoning is humbug, and not science!"

The human engine must first be seen before all other physiological considerations as an air-gas engine, constructed in its entirety—with the exception of the bones—from *rubber-like, very elastic, spongy material* called flesh and tissues.

The next fact is that its function is that of a pump system by air pressure, and with an inside circulation of liquids such as the blood and other saps, and that the lungs are the pump and the heart is the valve—and not the opposite—as erroneously taught by medical physiology for the past 400 years!

A further fact—one that has been almost entirely overlooked—is the automatic, atmospheric outside counter-pressure, which is over 14 pounds to the square inch. Immediately upon and after each out-breath, a vacuum is created in the lung cavity. In other words, the human body animal organism in its entirety functions automatically by inhaling air pressure, and expelling chemically changed air and outside atmospheric counter-pressure on the vacuums of the body. That is vitality, animal life in the first instance and importance.

46

That is "P" (power), which keeps you alive; and without air you cannot live five minutes.

But the unseen fact—let us say the secret, is that it works simply and automatically through atmospheric counter-pressure, which is only possible because the "engine" consists of elastic, spongy material with a vital strain power—with an ability of vibration, expansion, and contraction. Those two facts were the unknown secrets concerning the automatic function of "P" as the phenomena of vitality. The chemist Hensel[35] has proven through chemical physiological formulas that this special vital elasticity of the tissues is due to a lime-sugar combination.

The Latin word "spira" means first air, and then spirit: "The breath of God" is in fact first, good fresh air![36] It has been said that breathing is life, and it is true that you develop vitality—health—through physical and breathing exercises. It is also true that you can remove "O" (obstruction) by higher air pressure and counter-pressure in this way. It is true that you remove and eliminate obstructions of foreign matter by local and constitutional vibrations, consisting of all kinds of physical treatments. It is true that you eliminate disease matters and obstructions, and therefore relieve every kind of disease, through an artificial speeding of the circulation giving more "air-gas" and vibrating the tissues. You increase "P" (power) artificially for a certain time, but you decrease the vital ability of the function of counter-pressure, weakening the rubber-like elasticity of the tissues. In other words, you increase "P" but not "V." To the contrary, this is done, and can be done, only at the expense of "V." You know from experience what happens to a rubber band continually kept stretched or overexpanded. It loses its elasticity.

You relieve diseases, but you slowly lower vitality, particularly of the especially elastic and spongy important organs of lung, liver, kidney, etc. You relieve, but do not heal, diseases perfectly. You lower vitality, just so long as you loosen, remove, and eliminate obstructions exclusively through political means (agents) and just so long as you do not stop the supply—the taking in of waste, of obstruction—by wrong mucus-forming; that is, disease-building, unnatural foods, you lower vitality.

47

Would anyone attempt to clean an engine through a continually higher speed and shaking? No! You would first flush with a dissolving liquid and then change your fuel supply, should it be a steam engine, the obstructions through waste being caused through the coal only partly burning.

This involves the problem of dietetics, which culminates in the solution of these questions over its history: WHICH ARE THE BEST FOODS? Meaning, which foods give most energy, endurance, health, and increased vitality, or which foods are the basic cause of diseased conditions and growing old? What is the essence of life, of vitality, breathing exercise, activity—a perfect mind or right food?

My formula, the equation shown in the heading, gives the enlightening answer and solves the problem in its entire mystery. Decrease "O" first by decreasing quantities of food of all kinds, or even food entirely (fast), if conditions tell you. Second, stop—or decrease at least—by all means obstruction-causing, mucus-forming foods, and increase dissolving, eliminating, obstruction-removing foods and you increase "P," meaning a more unobstructed function of "P," of air pressure, of the infinite, inexhaustible power source. In other words, the problem of vitality and animal life functioning at all consists of unobstructed, perfect circulation by air pressure, and of a vital elasticity of the tissues through proper food as the necessary counter-pressure for the function of life.

"P" is infinite, unlimited, and practically the same everywhere and on everybody continually the same, but its activity slows down in the tempo (speed) as you accumulate obstructions, as you overeat and eat wrongly, lowering the automatic counter-pressure of the tissues.

You may now see that vitality does not depend immediately, directly, and primarily from food or from a right diet. If you eat too much of the best ones, especially in a body full of wastes and poisons, it is impossible for them to enter into your bloodstream in a clean state and become "efficiency-giving" vital substances. They are mixed with and poisoned by mucus and auto-toxemias, and actually lower vitality—they increase "O" instead of "P." You now see and you may realize very deeply, that it is worthless to figure food values with the intention of increasing "P" or "V" as long as the body is full of "O."

This problem is solved by my system, consisting of periodical minor fasting, alternating with cleansing, not nourishing, mucus-less and mucus-poor menus. Not as wrongly done with the idea that "V" is directly increased on a sick person through feeding clean food. Remove "O" through intelligent, personally prescribed menus. "P" increases automatically after a fast through its unobstructed function. You can now realize how wrong and insufficient it is for people to think that all there is to the "Mucusless Diet" is knowing the right foods!

Here then, is the cause why so many "fasting," "fruit diet," etc., "cures" fail. THE INEXPERIENCED LAYPERSON ALWAYS COMES TO THE DEATH POINT. In other words, he or she removes "O" too rapidly, too much at once, and feels "fine" for a while. The dissolving process goes deeper—"O" increases—they feel terribly weak, fall back on wrong diet, and thus this wrong diet stops the elimination of more obstructions, feels well again—blames the food for their weakness, and sees the wrong food as the food of vital efficiency. They lose their faith and tell you in all sincerity, "I have tried it, but it is wrong." They blame the system, entirely ignorant regarding it, when they alone are to blame. Here is the stumbling block even of other diet experts and naturopaths experimenting in dietetics. Lesson 7 will divulge this secret.

Some have had more experiences, but very few think as I do that Vitality, Energy and Strength are not derived from food at all! They believe it is acquired through sleep, etc. What I have learned and what I know through years of experimenting, and what I have actually demonstrated, can be found in my book, *Rational Fasting*, but briefly stated, it is this:

FIRST—Vitality does not descend primarily and directly from food, but rather from the facts of how far and how much the function of the human engine is obstructed—"braked" by obstructions of mucus and toxemias.

SECOND—Removing "O" by artificially increasing "P" and shaking, vibrating tissues through physical treatments is done at the expense of "V," Vitality.

THIRD—Vital energy, physical and mental efficiency, endurance, superior health by "P," air and water alone, are tremendous, beyond imagination—as soon as "P" works and can work without "O," without obstruction and friction, in a perfectly clean body.

FOURTH—the limit of going without food, and before solid food is necessary under such ideal conditions, is yet unknown.

FIFTH—the composition of "P" besides air, oxygen, and a certain quantity of water-steam, increases—but only in a clean body—by the following other agents from the infinite:

ELECTRICITY,

OZONE,

LIGHT (especially sunlight), and

ODOR (good smells of fruit and flowers)

Further, it is not impossible that under such clean, natural conditions, nitrogen of the air may be assimilated.

In the following lesson, I teach you a NEW but TRUE PHYSIOLOGY of the BODY, which is necessary to know in order to understand why and how the *MUCUSLESS DIET HEALING SYSTEM* works in its complete perfection, and for this purpose it was first necessary to lift the veil from the secret, FROM THE MYSTERY OF VITALITY.[37]

---

[35] Dr. Julius Hensel (1844-1903) was a pioneering agriculturalist, chemist, and author of *Bread from Stones and Life: Its Foundations and the Means for its Preservation; A Physical Explanation for the Practical Application of Agriculture, Forestry, Nutrition, the Functions of Life, Health and Disease and General Welfare*, the latter of which is quoted by Ehret in Lesson VIII of the *Mucusless Diet Healing System*.

[36] The word "spirit" is from the mid-thirteenth century, first meaning the "animating or vital principle in man and animals," the Old French *espirit*, and from Latin *spiritus* meaning "soul, courage, vigor, breath," related to *spirare* or *spiro*, meaning "to breathe."

[37] Ehret offers the equation Vitality = Power - Obstruction as an eloquent solution to the most injurious dietetic and physiological paradox in history: the belief that our body needs to consume so-called "nutritious" materials that will ultimately promote its death. He criticizes many commonly held theories of metabolism, protein, and nutrition, and offers new physiological explanations derived from experimenting with his mucus theory. Ehret's findings suggest that our bodies do not need to take in substances that cause illness to live, and that pus- and mucus-forming foods are the greatest proponents of human illness. Thus, the most fundamental human right is that we do not need to consume harmful, mucus-forming foods. In other words, we need not consume that which is unnecessary and damaging to human life. Instead of being obsessed with eating *nutritiously*, Ehret asserts that our focus should be on the most fundamental aspect of human life, which is breathing and the natural elimination of internal waste.

What is meant by V = P - O (Vitality = Power - Obstruction)? It is an equation devised by Ehret that he calls the "formula of life." Ehret's proposition is that the human body is a *perpetual motion air-gas engine* that is powered exclusively by oxygen and that the body ceases to function when obstructed with waste. He asserts that mucus-forming foods create obstruction in the human body, and that a diet consisting of starchless, fat-free fruits and green, leafy vegetables is the only diet that does not leave behind obstructive residues in the body and will aid the body in the process of natural healing. If these acidic obstructions are not able to be eliminated from the body, the deterioration of internal organs becomes almost inevitable.

If you were to put sand into the gas tank of your car, how far do you think your car would go? If your car engine is caked with gunk because you have not had the oil changed in years, how well does the car work? Chances are, it would work much better if gasoline was used instead of sand and the gunk (obstruction) was eliminated with a good oil change. If the basic laws are ignored, the obstruction in the engine becomes too great, and it cannot function and ultimately stops (dies). The engine of your body acts the same way. Your body is an air-gas engine that was never designed to take in mucus-forming foods. Over time, these mucus-forming foods create so much obstruction that your body can no longer receive efficient amounts of oxygen into the bloodstream. This obstruction is then given some name, such as heart attack, stroke, high cholesterol, etc.

To describe this basic principle, Ehret created the equation Vitality = Power - Obstruction, i.e., $V = P - O$. As soon as Obstruction (O) becomes greater than the body's Power (P) deriving from the breath, the body comes to a standstill.

It takes many people a great deal of time to truly understand Vitality = Power - Obstruction. It is very simple, yet elegant and profound. People often ask the difference between "vitality" and "power." More specifically, how "power" should be defined. Energy/vitality is the ability to do work; i.e., the more energy a device has, the more work it can do. Energy cannot be created or destroyed, but only changed or diverted. Power is the amount of work that can be done within a particular unit of time. Obstruction is the friction that prevents this work from functioning properly, therefore negatively impacting energy/vitality. In sum, energy/vitality is what is transferred, and power is the rate at which it is delivered.

In physics, power is the rate at which energy is transferred, used, or transformed. In this equation, Vitality may be likened to Energy, and Obstruction to Friction, i.e., Energy = Power - Friction. From Ehret's perspective, Power is the unknown constant and the rate of its transfer is based on the amount of friction afforded by an obstructing medium. Essentially, Vitality = Power would suggest that the human body is a perpetual motion air-gas machine that continues indefinitely without any external source of energy or change. In other words, the motion of a hypothetical machine that, once activated, would run indefinitely unless subject to an external force or to wear.

The New Physiology

Lesson VI

As you now know what Vitality is and how simply animal life functions automatically by air pressure and air counter-pressure (on fish, etc., it acts exactly the same, by water instead of air), you may realize that medical physiology, the science of animal functions, is fundamentally wrong based on the following errors which have to be corrected by a new physiology:

1. The theory of blood circulation,

2. Metabolism of the change of matter,

3. High protein foods,

4. Blood composition, and

5. Blood building.

The Error of Blood Circulation

Medical physiology, pathological physiology, continues to find diseases, i.e., the cause of disease, with the microscope, and germ theory is now "fashionable." They will never find the truth and never understand what disease is as long as they have a fundamentally wrong conception of blood circulation.

As I have already explained, the fact has been overlooked that the lungs are the motoric organs of circulation, and the circulating blood drives the heart—the same as the regulating valve in an engine. That the bloodstream drives the heart *and not the opposite* can be seen through the two following facts:

1. As soon as you increase air pressure by increased breathing, you speed the circulation and therefore the number of heart beats.

2. As soon as you take into the circulation a stimulating poison—alcohol for example—you *increase* the speed of the heart. As soon as you take a nerve and "muscle-band" paralyzing poison—for example, digitalis—you *decrease* the speed of the heart. The medical profession has this exact knowledge, but in spite of their knowledge, arrives at the *wrong conclusion* that a mysterious power acts on the heart muscle driving the blood circulation.

Prominent engineers among my patients agreed with my concept after learning this new physiology, saying that the heart would make a model valve for any kind of engine.

How can it be logically proven that the heart controls the circulation, if through the circulating blood you can control the heart?

Increased air pressure through climbing a hill or running increases heart action, for the speed of the valve, as in an engine, depends upon the pressure.

Thirty years ago, a Swiss expert of physiology, although a layperson, demonstrated evidentially with animal experiments that a circulation as taught by physiology, and as originated by Professor William Harvey[38] in London 400 years ago, does not exist at all. Of course, no attention was given by medicine to his demonstrations. How can a "science" be erroneous?

Metabolism

Metabolism, or the "science of the change of matter," is the most absurd and the most dangerous doctrine-teaching ever imposed on humankind. It is the father of the wrong cell theory and of that most erroneous, albumen theory,[39] which will kill and stamp out the entire

54

civilized Western world if its following is not stopped. It will kill you, too, someday, if you fail to accept the truth that a continual albumen replacement is *unnecessary*, and that you cannot gain vitality, efficiency, and health by protein as long as your human "engine" has to work *against* obstructions, which are in fact the cause of death of all humankind of the western civilization.

The erroneous idea that the cells of the body are continually used up by the process of life in their essential substance of protein and must be continually replaced by high protein foods can be and are evidentially refuted by my investigations, experiments, and observations on some hundred fasters. The facts are as follows, and you will again see that it is just as I teach and as I have experienced. What medicine calls and views as metabolism is the elimination of waste by the body as soon as the stomach is empty. Medicine actually believes that you live from your own flesh substance as soon as you are fasting. Even Dr. Kellogg[40] believed that the vegetarian becomes a meat eater when he or she fasts, and naturopathy has taken over, more or less, in principle these medical errors.[41] One believes that the human engine cannot run a minute without solid food, protein, and fat, and makes the erroneous conclusion that humans die and must die from starvation as soon as all their fat and protein is used up during a fast.[42] I found and have this to state:

Lean people can fast easier and longer than fat ones. The Hindu fakir, consisting of skin and bones, the leanest type in existence, can fast the longest time, and without suffering.[43] Where is there any "using up of the body" in this instance? I further found that the cleaner the body from waste (mucus) the easier and longer one can fast. Therefore a fast has to be prepared for by an eliminating and laxative diet. My world record of watched fasting of 49 days could be done under the conditions imposed only after using a strict mucusless diet during a long period of time. In other words, I could stand this long fast, and you can stand a fast much easier and much longer, the more the body is free from fat—which is partly decomposed, watery flesh—the more the body is free from mucus and poisons, which are eliminated as soon as eating is stopped, entirely or partly. The human body does not expel, burn up, or use up a single cell that is in vital condition! The cleaner—the freer from obstructions, from waste— the body is, the easier and the longer you can fast with water and air

55

alone! The limit where real starvation sets in is yet unknown! The Catholic Church claims tests of holy people who fasted during decades. But the medical error even grows by teaching metabolism, claiming that you must replace cells (which are not used up as you can plainly see) with high protein food from a cadaver, *partly decomposed meat*, and which has gone through a most destructive heat process of cooking! The fact is that you accumulate more or less of the wastes in your system in the shape of mucus and its poisons as the slowly growing foundation of your disease and the ultimate cause of your death. Human imagination is evidently not sufficient to conceive the tremendous foolishness of this doctrine and its consequences, unmindful that its teachings are actually said to kill the individual and to finally kill all humankind!

Medicine—and the average person, of course—also believes that you are growing flesh and increasing "good health," if you daily increase your weight by "good eating." If the colon of a so-called "healthy" fat man or woman is cleansed of their accumulated feces— even though they have "regular" stools, he or she at once loses from five to 10 pounds of the weight called "health."

Weight of feces, figured by doctors as health! Can you imagine anything more erroneous, more wrong, more foolish, and at the same time more dangerous to your health and life?

That is the medical "science" of metabolism.

---

[38] William Harvey (1578-1657) was an English physician and professor noted for being the first to completely describe the systemic circulation and properties of human blood in detail. However, earlier writers had provided precursors of the theory.

[39] The *albumen theory*, or *nitrogenous-albumin metabolic theory*, purports that humans must eat protein-rich, pus- and mucus-forming foods to provide fuel for, rebuild, and sustain the body.

[40] John Harvey Kellogg (1852–1943) was an American medical doctor in Battle Creek, Michigan, who ran a sanitarium using holistic methods with a particular focus on diet, enemas, and exercise. Kellogg was an advocate of

vegetarianism and is best known for the invention of the corn flakes breakfast cereal with his brother, Will Keith Kellogg.

[41] The term "vegetarian" refers to a variety of dietetic modalities that include the eating of plant-based foods (fruits and vegetables) and certain mucus-forming foods (starches or grains and fats). Some vegetarians may or may not also choose to include pus-forming foods such as dairy products, eggs, or fish.

[42] The "additive principle" is a term used by modern-day practitioners of the *Mucusless Diet Healing System* to refer to the belief that humans need to consume, accumulate, and use various forms of material matter to exist. Modern theories of nutrition and metabolism emerge from an additive concept, whereby it is thought that the human body must take in and metabolize various elements not obtained through the process of breathing to live. Ehret rejects the foundation of the additive principle and proposes his "formula to life" (Vitality = Power - Obstruction), which asserts that human life exists as a result of the non-accumulation, and elimination, of unnecessary matter. Therefore, emphasis is put on using food to help the body "eliminate" waste rather than obtaining "nutrition."

[43] A "fakir" is an ascetic mendicant or holy person, especially one who performs feats of endurance, rejects worldly pleasures, and lives solely on alms.

The New Physiology—Part 2

Lesson VII

High-Protein Foods

When the movement for naturopathy and a meatless diet began in the nineteenth century, medical scientists were endeavoring to prove by mathematical figures that physical and mental efficiency have to be kept up through daily replacement of protein, with a certain quantity for the average human. In other words, it became fashionable—a mania—to suggest and to do exactly the opposite of nature's laws whenever a person felt weak, tired rapidly, or became exhausted or sick in any way.[44]

You now know, through Lesson V, the source of Vitality and Efficiency. You also now know that the strength of a sick body can be increased when foods are not eaten, especially protein.

High protein foods act as stimulation for a certain time, because they decompose at once in the human body into poison. It is a commonly known fact that any kind of animal substance becomes very poisonous as soon as it enters into oxidation with air, especially at a higher temperature as exists in the human body.

59

The learned have gone so far as to prove that humans belong biologically in the class of meat-eating animals, while the descendant theory proves that they belong to the ape family, who are exclusively fruit eaters. You can see how ridiculous—contradictory—so-called "science" is.

The fundamental fact and truth of why the grown man or woman does not need so much protein as the old physiology claims is shown in the combination of mother's milk, which does not contain over two and a half to three percent protein, and nature builds up with that the foundation of a new body.

But the error goes further than that in their endeavor to replace something that is not destroyed, not used up, not "consumed" at all—as you learned in the previous lesson about the medical error of metabolism. The physiology has a principally wrong conception of change of matter, because these "experts," the founders of such a kind of science, lacked all knowledge of chemistry at all and organic chemistry especially. Life is based on change of matter in the meaning of physiological chemical transformation, but never on the absurd idea that you must eat protein to build, to grow, protein of muscles and tissue. Most certainly not; for instance, is it necessary that a cow must drink milk to produce milk?[45] A prominent expert of physiological chemistry, Dr. von Bunge, Professor of Physiological Chemistry at the University of Basel, Switzerland, whose books do not endorse the average standing of medical teaching, says that life, vitality, is based on transformation of substances (foods) through which power, heat, and electricity become free and act as efficiency in the animal body.

You will learn in the lesson about blood building that a certain change of matter happens in the human body, and how protein is produced through transformation from other food substances. This change of matter takes place not by replacement of old cells by new ones, but that mineral substances are the building blocks of animal and vegetable life, and the replacement is of much smaller quantities than as now taught.

The reason a "one-sided" meat eater can live a relatively longer time than the vegetarian "starch-eater" is easy to understand after having learned Lesson V. The first one produces less solid obstructions by smaller quantities of meat-foods than the starch "overeater," but their later diseases are more dangerous because they accumulate more poisons, pus, and uric acid.

If you know the truth about human nourishment—and you are going to learn it later—you will be amused to note how physiologists grope in darkness—how they made up a standard quantity of necessary albumen for the average human, which standard, by the way, is slowly getting smaller. They, and even advanced "diet experts," estimate without knowing the great unknown; i.e., the waste in the human body. For thousands of previous years, humans have lived healthier without food value formulas, and I doubt very much if a single one of these physiologists ever gave their "chef" a suggestion of food values.

The entire proposition is a farce, masquerading as a so-called science. A few, like Professor Chittenden,[46] found through experimenting that energy and endurance increased with less food—especially less protein. Professor Hindhede[47] proved that albumen need hardly be considered, and Fletcher[48] outdid them all. He lived on one sandwich a day curing his so-called "incurable" disease and developed a tremendous endurance.

After I had overcome all fear as to the fatal consequences that would befall me if I failed to adhere strictly to "scientific protein" necessities, I found, experienced, and demonstrated the hitherto unknown and unbelievable fact that in the clean, mucus-free, and poison-free body, these foods poorest in protein—fruits—develop the highest energy and an unbelievable endurance.

If nitrogen, the essential part of protein, is an important factor to keep the human machine running—if vitality depends at all on nitrogen, then it seems to me that under these ideal conditions nitrogen is assimilated from the air.

Food from the Infinite! "P" (power) as a source of nourishment! What tremendous possibilities! I suggest that you read Lesson V over again, and you will realize these two facts:

1. The truth about human nourishment is still a "book with seven seals"[49] to all humankind, all so-called diet experts and scientific experts included.

2. The error of high protein foods as a necessity of health, taught and suggested by medical doctrines to humankind, is in its consequences and in its effect just the opposite of what it should be; it is one of the main and general causes of all disease; it is the most tragic phenomena of western degeneration. It produced at the same time the most dangerous, most destructive habit of glutton; it produced the greatest madness ever imposed on humankind; that is, to endeavor to heal a disease by eating more, and especially more high-protein foods. It is beyond possibility to express in words what the error of high-protein foods means. Let me remind you that medicine claims as the father of medicine the great dietician Hippocrates, who said: "The more you feed a sick person, the more you harm him"; also: "Your food shall be your remedies, and your remedies your food."

When we allow the body to become clogged with mucus and other foreign obstructions such as calcium, phosphates, and similar waste materials, we may expect to have high blood pressure overburdening the heart in its efforts to keep the bloodstream circulating properly.

---

[44] Ehret refutes the notion of nutrition. From Ehret's perspective, the kind of attention that is paid to nutrition should be focused on the elimination of wastes from the body. The word "nutrition" (circa 1550) derives from L. nutritionem (nom. nutritio) meaning "a nourishing," from nutrire "nourish, [to] suckle." Here, we see that the original notion of nutrition had to do with nourishment, particularly that of a mother nursing her baby, i.e., to suckle ("nurse" is also related to "nourish"). Thus, the original concept of nutrition did not have to do with mathematical figures which seek to define the way in which elements must be replaced in the body. It was more of a natural concept connected to the means by which a person, especially an infant, sustains him or herself. From an Ehretist perspective, the primary purpose for an infant to consume their mother's milk is to slow down or aid in their own elimination. It may also be observed that infants initially consume only liquids and must be slowly transitioned into solid foods.

Contemplating this process may be helpful while learning the principles of the transition diet and fasting.

[45] This is a very important statement, as it simply and elegantly shows how wrong it is to think that we must eat dead animal flesh, or drink animal milk, to create human flesh. What cow needs to drink milk to produce milk? What cow eats dead animal flesh to produce its own beef? Cows are herbivores and will eat only grass if in the proper environment. Also, many primates will live on fruits only, or fruits and herbs, if in the correct environment. Many of these animals are not small, weak, or deficient in any way.

[46] Russell Henry Chittenden (1856-1943) was an American physiological chemist and professor. He is known for having conducted pioneering research in the biochemistry of digestion and was a founding member of the American Physiological Society in 1887.

[47] Mikkel Hindhede (1862-1945) was a Danish physician and nutritionist, born on the farm Hindhede outside Ringkøbing on the Danish west coast. He was the manager of the Danish National Laboratory for Nutrition Research in Copenhagen 1910-1932 and food advisor to the Danish government during World War I. In his research, he challenged prevailing theories about the amount of protein humans need to eat, and as a practitioner, he recommended eating less meat and more plant-based foods.

[48] Horace Fletcher (1849-1919) was an American health food enthusiast of the Victorian era nicknamed "The Great Masticator" from his strong arguments that every bite must be chewed about 100 times per minute before being swallowed. He and his supporters advocated the practice of "Fletcherizing," that is, chewing each bite numerous times, as well as a low-protein diet. See Ehret's discussion of FLETCHERISM.

[49] "Book with seven seals" is a phrase that refers to or suggests some kind of secret (esoteric) knowledge that is not easily accessible or understood by humans. "Seven seals" is a phrase originally used in the Book of Revelation of the Bible which refers to seven symbolic seals that secure the book, or scroll, that John of Patmos saw in his Revelation of Jesus Christ. The opening of the seals of the Apocalyptic document occurs in Revelation Chapters 5-8.

The New Physiology—Part 3

Lesson VIII

Blood Composition

The logical consequence of the first three errors of the Old Physiology is the problem of composition of human blood as not only what it should be but also as a fact of "scientific examination." The error is so great that it borders on insanity.

The problem is this: Are the white corpuscles living cells of vital importance to protect and maintain life, to destroy germs of disease, and to immunize the body against fever, infection, etc., as the standard doctrines of physiology and pathology teach?

Or, are they just the opposite—waste, decayed, undigested, unusable food substances, mucus, pathogens, as Dr. Thomas Powell calls them?[50] They are indigestible by the human body, unnatural, and therefore not assimilated at all. Are they, in fact, the waste from high-protein and starchy foods which the average mixed eater of western civilization stuffs in their stomach three times a day? Is what I call "mucus" the foundational cause of all diseases?

Pathology proves that by saying that the white corpuscles are increased in case of disease and physiology says they increase during digestion in the healthy body, and that they are derived from high-protein foods.

65

This teaching is absolutely correct, and the logical consequence of the error of high-protein foods.

Medical "science" sees and must see it as normal conditions of health, and that the non-sick must have these white blood corpuscles in their circulation because everybody has them. There is no person in existence in the western civilization whose body has not been continually stuffed since childhood with cow milk, meat, eggs, potatoes, and cereal products. No person today without mucus!

In my first published article, I promulgated the gigantic idea that the white race is an unnatural, a sick, and a pathological one. First, the colored skin pigment is lacking in coloring mineral salts; second, the blood is continually overfilled by white blood corpuscles, mucus, and waste with white color. This is the reason for the white appearance of the entire body.[51]

The skin pores of the white people are constipated by white, dry mucus—their entire tissue system is filled up and filled out with it. No wonder that they look white and pale and anemic. Everybody knows that an extreme case of paleness is a "bad sign." When I appeared with my friend in a public air bath, after having lived for several months on a mucusless diet with sun baths, we looked like Indians and people believed that we belonged to another race. This condition was doubtless due to the great amount of red blood corpuscles and the great lack of white blood corpuscles. I can notice a trace of paleness in my complexion the morning after eating one piece of bread.

This is not the place to bring up all of the arguments against this terrible error about the nature and "function" of the white blood corpuscles believed erroneously by medical "science." Any one desiring a real scientific proof of this may read Dr. Thomas Powell's *Fundamentals and Requirements of Health and Disease*, published in 1909—a few years after my "mucus theory" was published in Europe, and later translated into English in 1913 as *Rational Fasting and Regeneration Diet*, neither of us knowing anything regarding each other's publication. Dr. Powell teaches in principal the same as I do, so far as the cause of all diseases, the white corpuscles, and all these medical errors are concerned. The only difference being that he calls "pathogen" what I call "mucus."

In the method of elimination and diet, however, I differ principally and entirely from him; but even in the composition of the red blood corpuscles, the blood plasma at all, the blood serum, and the so-called hemoglobin, medical "science" lacks perfection.

The two most important facts for us to know are these:

1. The first is the much greater importance and vital necessity of iron in the human body.

2. The second is the presence of sugar-stuff in the blood. The great expert of physiological chemistry and mineral salts theory founder, Hensel, says in his book *Life*, "Iron is chemically veiled in our blood." Doctors could not find it through their lack of knowledge in chemistry. On page 36 of the same book, he says, "In our blood albumen is a combination of sugar-stuff and iron oxide, but not to be found or recognized (discovered) in such a way that neither the sugar nor the iron can be found by ordinary chemical tests. The blood albumen must be burned first to make the test perfect."

I presume that the truth and importance is this: The red color of blood is the most characteristic quality of this "quite special sap" and is due to iron oxide, rust![52] Therefore, it is self-evident how important iron is in the blood. Further—the sugar stuff is of high importance besides its nourishing quality, as it is an essential part in the perfect blood hemoglobin, which if in a perfect state has to become thick, like gelatin, as soon as it comes in contact with the atmospheric air for the purpose of closing a wound. Read in my book *Rational Fasting* my test of a nonbleeding, immediate healing wound, without secretion of pus and mucus, without pain and inflammation.

One truth regarding the conditions of the human blood found out by doctors is that acidity is a sign of disease. It is no small wonder that this readily happens with the mixed eater, when they fill the stomach daily with meat, starch, sweets, fruits, etc., all at the same time.

Make a personal test if you are not fully convinced. Eat a regular dinner, and one hour after eating, get it out of your stomach and you will have a sour fermenting mixture of a terrible odor, reminding you of the garbage pail, and which when fed to hogs causes even these animals to slowly become sick.

Or, if you do not care to be so heroic, try the following experiment: Next time you sit down to your Sunday dinner, have the menu served for an imaginary guest. Empty their portion in a cooking vessel, using the same quantities as you are eating and drinking yourself. Stir thoroughly. Then cook on an oven at blood heat for not less than 30 minutes. Place a cover on the vessel and leave overnight. When you remove the cover in the morning, a distinct surprise will await you.

---

[50] In the late nineteenth and early twentieth centuries, a surge of medical researchers whose evidence challenged the newly developed theories of protein and albuminous foods emerged. In his book entitled *Fundamentals and Requirements of Health and Disease* (1909), Dr. Thomas Powell, MD challenges what he calls the "Nitrogenous Food Theory." He states "this theory has enjoyed a long season of popularity and yet it is an undeniable fact that the notion that nitrogen is the prime essential of food is wholly fallacious, having no other foundation than an erroneous supposition and a misinterpretation of facts—errors which have led to a desperate misuse or abuse of the most valuable of all foods" (Powell, 41). He goes on to challenge the germ theory and asserts that albuminous foods play the most important role in most human illness. "The biologic, physiologic and much of the dietetic and pathological teaching of this day and age is founded upon the assumptions that the 'white blood corpuscle' is a 'living cell'; that it is 'differentiated' into the tissues of the body; that it is a 'phagocyte' or germ-devourer and that the material in which it is found and from which it is formed . . . is the 'physical basis of life'" (Powell, 263). He then asks the following question:

> Is it not entirely reasonable to suppose that the motility of
> the white blood corpuscle is due to the forces not of life,
> but of death; to the processes not of vital duplication, but
> of chemical dissolution—that is, to the combined effects

of chemotaxis, disintegration and gaseous expansion . . . ?
(Powell, 275)

Powell's argument parallels Ehret's by asserting that the leukocyte (white corpuscle) is "not a living cell, but a particle of dead and perishable material" (Powell, 292). He adds that "the irony of the situation into which the leukocyte addendum to the cell-theory has led us is not only perfectly discernible, but as cruel and relentless as the grave, since it is to the effect that the more 'tissue-building' material (white corpuscles) the sick person carries in his circulation, that more pronounced is his debility and emaciation, and that the more 'vigilant policeman' (phagocytes) he has to guard and defend him, that more certain and speedy is his destruction" (Powell, 294). (For further reading please see Powell, "The Cell-Theory," in *Fundamentals and Requirements of Health and Disease* 263-294).

[51] Ehret's proposition is that skin color and other physiological traits primarily reflect the degree to which a person is internally encumbered with waste on the cellular level. It challenges the popular notion that the radical physical morphology of humans occurred based primarily on adapting to non-tropical climates further away from the equator.

[52] To understand this statement, it is important to consider the role of iron in the blood. When iron that is mined from the earth comes into contact with oxygen, dark rust is produced (iron-oxide). When our blood iron comes into contact with air, i.e. oxygen, it also rusts. Clean blood that is free of waste easily rusts when oxidized. To demonstrate this argument, Ehret tells of his experiments with self-inflicted bleeding. He found that when he ate a mucusless diet for an extended period of time, a knife wound would heal immediately with no secretion of pus and mucus. He would also suffer no pain or inflammation. Thus, the oxygen would mix with the iron in the blood and rust immediately. However, when he ate mucus-forming foods, his wounds did not easily heal, and he suffered from pain. He also became paler. This experiment suggests that 1) a mucusless diet promotes clean blood, 2) clean blood is free of white waste materials, and 3) clean blood becomes darker when oxidized. Given that blood becomes dark when mixed with oxygen on the outside of the body, to what extent does this happen inside the body? When clean blood is oxidized through the act of breathing, can it *rust* and darken? Hensel's argument may shed some light on these questions: "In our blood albumen is a combination of sugar-stuff and iron oxide, but not to be found or recognized (discovered) in such a way that neither the sugar nor the iron can be found by ordinary chemical

tests. The blood albumen must be burned first to make the test perfect" [Ehret summarizing Hensel's *Life*, Lesson 8]. Consequently, the red color of blood is due to iron-oxide, i.e. rust. Furthermore, the ability for red blood to become oxidized is dependent upon the absence of albumen, i.e. mucus/waste.

Ehret's perspectives on the nature of blood are controversial and challenging. But, one does not need to initially believe in them to benefit from practicing the mucusless diet. Ehret offers a fresh perspective, and it is important to keep an open mind as you move forward. It is helpful to remember that Ehret is a masterful philosopher of diet and physiology. As a philosopher, Ehret's work questions and challenges the very foundation of Western dietetic theory and physiological science. Yet, in order to truly understand many of these concepts, it will be important to practice and experience the diet. Much of what Ehret discusses tends to become self-evident through a dedicated adherence to his dietetic principles.

The New Physiology—Part 4

Lesson IX

Blood Building

The problem of blood building in the human body involves all problems of health and disease. In other words, your health and disease depend almost entirely on your diet; whether you eat right or wrong foods, which foods harm you, thereby building and producing disease, and which foods heal and keep your body in ideal condition; which ones build natural, good blood and which ones build wrong, bad, acid, diseased blood?[53] These questions and their correct answers are the fundamentals of dietetics and of my *Mucusless Diet Healing System*. In this lesson, I teach only the principal truth in general. All particulars and details are covered in the entire course.

In fact, my diet of healing in its main and essential part consists of building a new, perfect blood with continual "supply" from natural foods with vital elements through which the bloodstream is enabled to dissolve and eliminate all waste, all mucus, all poisons, and all drugs ever taken during a lifetime, wherever and for as long a time as they may have been "stored up" as latent disease in the body.

What the "official" physiology of nourishment teaches for best blood building is doubly wrong. First, it is wrong principally as a problem of physiological chemistry and second, from the truth of nature.

Here again I must quote that great authority of physiological chemistry, Prof. von Bunge, who personally told me that he does not endorse official, medical teaching. Says von Bunge, "Life is based on transformation of substances, through which process power, efficiency, becomes free, just as it takes place in every chemical process of transformation from one chemical entity of atoms and molecules into another one."

The authors that started physiological science lacked, principally, knowledge in chemistry due to a more humanistic education rather than in science of nature. On the other hand, inorganic chemistry was not sufficiently developed at this time.

The misleading idea was again protein. They reasoned as follows: Muscles, tissues, the entire body's essential substance is protein—therefore, this substance must be introduced into the blood in order to build, to grow—in other words, you must eat muscles to build muscles, you must eat protein to build protein, you must eat fat to build fat, and in the case of a nursing mother, she must drink milk to make milk!

As they believed and still believe in metabolism and the necessity of replacing every day used-up cells, these principles are followed in the diet of the average mixed eater.

To take an inorganic iron, lime, etc., in an endeavor to replace the same substance in the body is a similar error.

The cow builds flesh, tissues, bones, hair, milk, efficiency, and heat, all from grass exclusively. Feeding milk to a cow to increase milk production would be classed as the height of folly, and yet humans do this very thing with themselves!

Today, every substance of the human body is chemically analyzed and doctors dream of perfecting chemically concentrated food substances in the future, making it possible for you to carry your meals in your vest pocket in sufficient quantities to last a couple of days. That will never happen for the human body, as it does not assimilate a single atom of any food substance that is not derived from the vegetable or fruit kingdom.

72

All manufactured food mixtures, when too concentrated—either of the animal or vegetable kingdom—does not build blood but stimulate only.[54]

Animal foods cannot build good blood; in fact, they do not build human blood at all, because of the biological fact that humans are by nature fruit eaters. Look at the juice of a ripe blackberry, black cherry, or black grapes. Doesn't it almost resemble your blood? Can any reasonable person prove that half-decayed "muscle tissues" build better blood?

Just as soon as the animal is killed, that flesh is more or less in decomposition. Then they are put through the destructive process of cooking. No meat-eating animal can live on cooked meat; they must eat it fresh and raw—blood, bones, and all.

Complete details about the right and natural foods will be taught later, and you will learn the truth. I will only mention at this time one important fact, which is essential in my dietetic teaching, and by which I differ from all others, even from other dietetic experts who still believe in concentrated albumen, concentrated mineral salts, etc., being required for good blood building.

Albumen is not the most important substance for our blood, nor is it mineral salts alone that build perfect blood. *THE CARDINAL STANDARD SUBSTANCE FOR HUMAN BLOOD IS THE HIGHEST DEVELOPED FORM OF CARBON HYDRATE, CHEMICALLY CALLED SUGAR-STUFF, GRAPE OR FRUIT SUGAR AS CONTAINED MORE OR LESS IN ALL RIPE FRUITS, AND IN THE NEXT LOWER STATE IN VEGETABLES.*[55] The newer advanced science teaches that even the small amount of protein that is necessary is developed from grape sugar. Vegetable-eating animals transform these foods, first into grape sugar, and then as a matter of fact, the body in its entirety.

But the essential point of disagreement regarding this particular problem is not in the food, blood-building problem. Whoever does not know disease—latent, acute, and chronic as taught in Lesson V, will never believe in the truth of human nourishment.

As you now know through past lessons, just as soon as the blood is improved through fruits, the average person immediately starts the elimination of obstructions—feels better for a while, but when more and more waste is dissolved and with the resultant next shock of obstruction in the circulation, all faith is lost, and they, the doctor, and all, blame the lack of "efficiency" food. They think, and every one suggests, that they need "regular food," which stimulates them for a while and causes them to believe that it must be the meat and eggs that build good blood.

In other words, the problem of blood building through right and proper food, the dietetic problem in its entirety will not be solved, and the truth will not be accepted nor believed and practiced by those who have not learned what happens, and just what it means to heal by the new and real blood-building foods.

This is the deeper reason why doctors believe in and recommend destructive foods, and why the average person keeps them up and increases them continually, for they do not possess the slightest idea of what disease is, and how they pollute their blood on a daily basis.

---

[53] In other words, your health and the diseases you suffer depend almost entirely on your diet. The wrong foods harm you and produce disease, while the right foods heal you and keep your body in an ideal condition through building natural, good blood. The harmful foods build wrong, bad, acidic, diseased blood.

[54] Stimulation means to temporarily increase the activity of an organism or its body organ. Ehret's proposition is that mucus-forming foods are not nurturing or "nutritious," but serve only to unnaturally stimulate the body like a poisonous drug.

[55] "Carbon hydrates," more commonly referred to as carbohydrates, are any of a large class of organic compounds consisting of carbon, hydrogen, and oxygen. They are produced in green plants by photosynthesis. Sugars, starches, and cellulose are all carbohydrates. For Ehret, the highest forms of carbohydrate-containing foods for humans are fresh, fat-free fruits derived of simple sugars.

74

Critique of all Other Healing Systems

And Unbiased, Unprejudiced Reviews

Lesson X

The methods of healing are numberless. Outside of a great domination of superstition in this field, the serious methods can be divided into two principally different classes:

1—MEDICINE

2—DRUGLESS HEALING

The history of medicine shows that, especially in the past, drugs and other mysterious "inventions" were taken from "quacks." A great number of "medicines," "standard remedies," for example, mercury, were introduced by "quacks." The modern serums, etc., are not better, regardless of their being "scientifically" prepared.

As we now know exactly what disease is, we may understand a fact medicine cannot explain, and that is *WHY* symptoms of disease can be suppressed by drugs and serums to a certain limit. The "results" are known only through experiences, but medicine does not know why these results—"special effects"—happen.

THIS IS THE SECRET: If the body of any sick person endeavors to eliminate poisons manifested by any kind of symptoms, and a new and dangerous poison is introduced into the circulation, that elimination through the symptoms is more or less stopped because the body instinctively sets to work to neutralize these poisons as far as it is possible. The symptoms return just as soon as the life is saved, and the same procedure is repeated until the patient dies—or if intelligent enough—casts medicine aside in time and seeks to save himself by DRUGLESS HEALING.

The methods of drugless healing are also very numerous, and they can be divided into three parts:

1. Physical treatments,

2. Mental treatments, and

3. Dietetic treatments.

Physical Treatments:

In general, all physical treatments have a tendency to loosen local constitutional encumbrances through various kinds of vibrations and thermal differences. The Kneipp cure, for instance, is in fact an application of artificial colds which stimulates the circulation, and through that, the elimination.

Exercise (calisthenics), breathing exercises, massage, osteopathy, physical therapy, etc., perform in principle the same. However, chiropractic claims a special "scheme." The subluxation is removed, but chiropractics, similarly to drugs, may give immediate successful relief from painful symptoms; but as a matter of fact they return sooner or later if the adjustments are discontinued and wrong method of living is persisted in. The cause of subluxation is an accumulation of foreign matters between the bones of the spine, and we know that they have their source through wrong eating, the same as all other symptoms of disease. No doubt the overweight of the average human, in general, is another cause of subluxation. Under longer fastings, I saw many deformed spines improve wonderfully.

There are various other methods used to shake the tissues and stimulate circulation, i.e., electricity, electric light, sunlight, etc. All of these methods help and relieve, more or less, but they can never heal perfectly just as long as they fail to pay sufficient attention to a correct diet. In other words, the elimination of disease or foreign

76

matters will never be complete as long as the intake through wrong foods is not discontinued and an entirely new blood building is established through real, natural, and clean, mucusless foods.

Mental Treatments:

It cannot be denied that the condition of the mind has an influence on every kind of disease. It is proven that fear, sorrows, and worries have a bad influence not only on the heart and nerves, but on the circulation, digestion, etc. Psychotherapy, mental and divine healing, Christian Science, have this one great advantage—they save the unfortunate sick from the injuries of drugs! On the other hand, I cannot grant them too much credit, for while they are harmless in a certain sense—they have a tendency, consciously or unconsciously, to keep people in complete darkness as to what disease really is.

We who know exactly what disease is cannot agree with a teaching that endeavors to make sick people believe they can be healed by a miracle or a forced imagination—that they are not sick at all—even though they are actually dying that very minute! It is farcical, not to say pitiful, to pray to the Creator for a miraculous healing—rejecting and disregarding real divine foods—the fruits of the paradise—the "bread of heaven," and instead stuff your stomach three times daily with harmful prepared foods, manufactured by humans for commercial purposes, and never designed by the Creator to be human's food at all.

It is rather difficult to believe in mental healing at all, after knowing as I do through actual experiences with thousands of patients that the average chronic sick, especially the well fed one, is in fact a "living cesspool." Nature is the manifestation of the divine laws, and *there are no miracles in Nature*. If you have eaten wrong for 30, 40, 50 years, thereby producing your disease, *you must do the necessary compensation* as reparation for your sins; you must do the opposite by eating clean, natural, divine food, which will produce health instead of disease. That is as clear as sunlight, and as logical as 2 x 2 = 4.

The philosophy of Mrs. Eddy is a poor copy of Schopenhauer's "World of Imagination"—that the mind only is real, and not the physical.[56] Her logic would be correct if she had said: "*It was never the intention, nor in the plan of God, to produce disease. But as a logical consequence, through disobedience of the divine laws of life, disease is produced.*" There could

77

be no disease if humans lived right in accordance with the divine story of the Genesis arguments.[57] In the light of evolution, we may understand the true meaning of the Lord, even when He says He "will punish and kill them till they come back to Him." In plain, instead of mysterious words, you and all humankind will suffer and die from disease so long as you fail to return again to the laws of the Creator, to the laws of Nature, as humans lived in paradise.

Practitioners of the *Mucusless Diet Healing System* should avail themselves of the knowledge already gained and live on mucusless foods, the divine clean food of Genesis, fruits and green-leaf vegetables (called herbs), so that they may demonstrate the truth as living examples. This will aid the patient to learn and believe the truth as exemplified by you, and free their mind from all wrong and superstitious ideas about disease, as well as from all doubts about the one and *only* way of real help, the compensation of their disease-producing habits.

You must heal, that is free, the patient's brain from all ignorance and lift their mind with the light of truth so that they may have unshaken faith to follow your advice with enthusiasm! That is the true essential for "mental healing."

---

[56] Mrs. Mary Baker Eddy (1821–1910) was the founder of Christian Science (1879), a controversial system of religious thought and practice adopted by the Church of Christ, Scientist. She was the author of the movement's textbook, *Science and Health with Key to the Scriptures*, and the founder of the Christian Science Publishing Society in 1898, which continues to publish a number of periodicals including *The Christian Science Monitor* (1908).

[57] See discussion of Genesis 1:29 in the notes of Lesson I.

Confusion in Dietetics

Lesson XI

In this very important lesson, it is necessary for me to convince you, once and for all, of the following facts:

FIRST—that in food (in diet) lies 99.99 percent of the causes of all diseases and imperfect health of any kind.

SECOND—that consequently, all healing, all therapeutics, will continue to fail so long as they refuse to place the most important stress on diet.

THIRD—that what I call "mucusless diet" and "mucus-forming foods" divides characteristically all human foods into harmless, natural, healing, and real nourishing foods—and into harmful, disease-producing ones.

FOURTH—that all other dietetics are mainly wrong because they lay their stress on food values entirely, whether "wrong" or not, instead of the healing, cleaning, eliminating values, and their efficiency before the healing process is started, going on, or accomplished at all. (See Lesson V)

The dietetic problem, "What shall humans eat to be healthy or to heal their disease," is, in fact, the problem of life—as little as it is considered or even known as the most important question. Long ago,

79

I coined the following phrase, "Life is a tragedy of nutrition."[58] The confusion and ignorance regarding what to eat is, in fact, so great that it must be necessarily called the "missing link" of the human mind.

That medical science and even so-called "natural" therapeutics see dietetics in general as a secondary question of healing is significant. Even the efficiency of a machine depends upon the quality and amount of its fuel. There is no longer any doubt existing regarding the fact that a plant depends more on the kind of soil rather than climate to produce a high-quality fruit. Farmers understand thoroughly that everything depends on what they feed their livestock. Health and disease of the animal and human body is 99.99 percent dependent on food. This is tremendously manifested by nature through the simple fact that every animal refuses food when sick. The animal instinct of responding to every disease or even accident by fasting is nature's demonstration that health and disease depend mainly and entirely from eating or not eating, as well as the kind of foods.

That the average person, and even the reformed doctors, blames everything on earth, excepting food, as the cause of their disease is due to the tragic fact that disease is as yet a mystery in their minds. They don't know how terribly unclean the inside of the body is caused through the life-long habit of overeating 10 times as much as required—in many cases harmful foods mostly, or even exclusively.

If the average eater, even in so-called "perfect health," fasts 3 or 4 days, their breath and the entire body as well as their discharges are of an offensive odor which signifies, demonstrates, and indicates that his or her system is filled up with decayed, uneliminated substances brought in through no other manner than by eating. This accumulated and continually increasing waste is his or her latent, unknown "disease," and when nature wants to eliminate it by any kind of a "shock," commonly known as disease, they first try everything to "heal" themselves excepting to fast, to *stop increasing* the cause of the disease—the inside waste.

You have now learned how wrong medicine is, trying to *stop* nature's healing, eliminating process, called disease, and thereby increasing the inside waste through drugs and serums. But "natural" therapeutics of all kinds of elimination will never heal perfectly just

80

so long as you fail to discontinue the supply of inside waste caused by eating and "wrong" eating. You may clean, and continue to clean indefinitely, but never with complete results up to a perfect cleanliness, as long as the intake of wrong or even *too much right foods* is not stopped.

If it is a fact that food alone is chiefly to blame for all disease—as nature so clearly demonstrates—then it is logical and self-evident that you can heal only by diet; and radically only, if necessary, with the most rational diet—fasting—nature's only "remedy" in the animal kingdom.

Therefore, if any kind of diet shall heal, it must consist of food not according to food values as to their nourishing and rebuilding qualities, but according to qualities of healing, of cleaning, and of elimination.

Here is the cardinal reason why, as well as where, all other dietetics fail. My diet of healing, the mucusless diet, divides, as stated above, all foods strictly into two kinds: certain ones which heal and certain ones which produce disease.

It is not sufficient, as the layperson imagines, to only know which foods are mucusless and which are mucus-forming, but:

1. HOW FAR AND HOW FAST THE CHANGE CAN SUCCESSFULLY BE MADE,

2. HOW THE COMBINATION OF DIFFERENT FOODS HAS TO BE ARRANGED, and

3. HOW LONG AND HOW OFTEN FASTING MUST BE INTRODUCED AND COMBINED DURING THE HEALING DIET IF FOUND NECESSARY.

This is the *SYSTEM* of the *Mucusless Diet* and *Fasting*. It represents what *THE PRACTITIONER HAS TO STUDY AND MUST LEARN*, and what the layperson does not know, and consequently why they must inevitably fail when trying to cure a person with "good foods."

After the foregoing explanation, you will at once see in the following critique of the best known dietetics why they are imperfect and why the confusion is so great. In later lessons, you will also learn of every kind of food, why it is good, and why bad. In case you are still unaware which of the foods are mucusless and which mucus-forming, they are as follows:

All fruits, raw or cooked; also nuts and green-leaf vegetables are mucus-free.[59]

All other foods of civilization, *without exception*, are mucus and acid-forming, and therefore are harmful.

---

[58] The meaning of Ehret's statement "a tragedy of nutrition" is often misunderstood, especially by those not familiar with his work. Many assume that Ehret is suggesting that the *tragedy* refers to the idea that people are not getting enough, or the right kind of, nutrition. But, as articulated in previous chapters, Ehret denounces what has become the traditional Western dietetic theory of nutrition. If Ehret does not support most concepts of "nutrition," then what does he mean by a "tragedy of nutrition"? Historically, the word *tragedy* initially referred to a play or other serious literary works with an unhappy ending. Later, it also came to be used to identify any unhappy event or disaster. My proposition is that the "tragedy of nutrition" is not about the lack, or poor choice of, nutritious foods. The tragedy is that the concept of nutrition 1) erroneously exists, and 2) is dietetically opposed to the truth of natural laws governing animal life on earth. In other words, the tragedy is not only that people eat poorly and die, but think that they are eating healthy, or taking drugs responsibly, and die not realizing that pus, mucus-forming foods, and drugs are the foundation of their demise. Nutrition is the great scientific paradox of our time, insofar as its doctrines teach that we must eat certain mucus-forming foods to survive, yet mucus-forming foods are not only unnatural for humans, but the foundation of human illness. For more of my thoughts on the concept of nutrition, see *Spira Speaks*.

[59] This statement often raises questions about what foods are, and are not, truly mucus-forming. First, the assertion that nuts are mucus-free contradicts what is said later in the book, when they are identified to be mucus-forming. Also, many readers assume that avocados are mucus-free because they are technically a "fruit." Although avocados are not addressed specifically by Ehret—as they did not become a prevalent salad item until the 1950s—Ehret's discussion about nuts can help us to understand the mucus-forming nature of avocados and other fatty fruits or vegetables. With that said, the mucusless diet does contradict itself regarding nuts.

In Lesson XVI on the Transition Diet, Ehret writes, "Other kinds of grated nuts or nut butter may be served once in a while for this purpose (transition diet), but are too rich in protein and will produce, if continually used, mucus and uric acid." In Lesson XXII "Destructive Diet of Civilization," he explains

> All nuts are too rich in protein and fat and should be eaten only in winter, and then only sparingly. Nuts should be chewed together with some dried sweet fruits or honey, never with juicy fruits, because water and fat do not mix.

With the possible exception of nuts, the above represent about all of the foods which have to be prepared in some manner for eating; in fact they are tasteless unless specially prepared (Lesson XXII).

The contradiction arises when Ehret asserts, "All fruits, raw or cooked; also nuts and green-leaf vegetables are mucus-free" (Lesson XI). To be clear, nuts are mucus-forming. But why was this statement made? There are several explanations for this, but the two main ones are that 1) in comparison with meat, nuts are virtually mucus-free, and 2) that Ehret's editor Fred Hirsch took certain liberties during the assemblage of early editions of the *Mucusless Diet* and may be responsible for the mishap. Some of these changes, or contributions, can be easily identified, as we will see later in the "Vegetarian Recipes" section, whereby the editor, obviously Hirsch, explains why he added the mucus-lean menus, although Ehret resisted requests to do so.

Ehret ultimately asserts that:

> Fats of any kind, including the ordinary butter, are unnatural and therefore should not be eaten (Lesson XV).

> All fats are acid forming, even those of vegetable origin, and are not used by the body. You will like, crave and use them only as long as you can still see mucus in the "Magic Mirror" (Lesson XXII).

This principle extends to all fatty fruits or vegetables, including avocados, nuts, coconut meat, olives, durian, etc.

Confusion in Dietetics—Part 2

Lesson XII

The average vegetarian diet omits only meat from the menu, and their mixture of larger quantities of fruits (good foods) with eggs and milk cause overeating—in most cases being worse than moderate meat eating, and a "less mixed" diet.

Three prominent physicians improved the vegetarian diet, but they fail like all other dieticians on the following single point. They believe, more or less, in high-protein foods during the diet of healing. In other words—all dieticians, without a single exception outside of myself, think that the body, and especially the sick and weak one, requires "good, nourishing food" to be healed—overlooking the fact that nature alone heals and does it best by fasting. (Please read Lesson V again, so that you may fully comprehend the reason.)

Dr. Lahmann, a German physician, proved in his "The Dietetical Disformation of Blood" that carbonic acid is the cause of all diseases—but he failed to see the deeper cause, the fermentation caused through mucus-forming foods mixed with fruits. He believed in—and fell a victim to—the protein theory, in spite of his greatly advanced knowledge.

Dr. Haig, an English physician, with his "Anti-uric-acid Diet" showed much improvement, but failed in the same manner as Dr. Lahmann.

Dr. Catani, an Italian physician, made up a diet of fruits, green vegetables, and meat, eliminating all starch, and healed, more or less, including cases of rheumatism and gout, which Dr. Haig blamed meat solely for these diseases. The secret of Dr. Catani's starchless diet is its laxative effect. It relieves like the laxatives contained in mineral-water springs, but does not heal perfectly. You can see where the point of confusion lies.

Dr. S. Graham, an American physician, whose "Physiology of Nourishment" was fundamental at the time—improved the bread especially; but the improvement consists not in the fact that graham, bran and whole wheat bread is more valuable than ordinary white bread, but through its efficiency owing to a less constipating quality than white bread. White flour *makes good paste*, graham, or whole wheat flour does not. Dr. Graham found an opponent in Dr. Densmore of England, who claimed that overeating of bran, whole cereals, and graham bread caused inflammation of the intestines. [60] This is, of course, an exaggeration, but Dr. Densmore helped the general improvement of dietetics by advocating more fruits and vegetables.

Dr. Lahmann, the German chemist Hensel, and some authorities in the United States are the founders of what may be called "the mineral salt" movement. The stress in this dietetic reasoning is placed upon the fact that all acid and mucus-forming foods lack the necessary mineral salts. But it proved a fad, like the protein fad, thinking health could be regained by overflowing the body with artificially manufactured mineral-salts preparations and keeping up your old wrong habits at the same time. You improve—relieve to a certain limit—but never heal perfectly. In a later lesson, you will learn how the chemist Ragnar Berg improved this "system" to a certain degree. A person neutralizes acid-forming foods with mineral-salt-rich ones.

Raw Food Diet

At present among the vegetarian health-seekers, "raw-food diet" is in fashion.[61] No doubt it represents great progress, but the arguments are partly wrong and lead to mistaken and fanatic extremes.

They claim all cooking destroys food values, but it should be said properly: "Wrong cooking destroys HEALING value qualities (efficiency) of foods and can even cause them to become acid forming." The "raw food" experts hint on the same wrong stress as all others, i.e., the higher food value.

The entire effect or benefit from raw food is the rough fiber of uncooked vegetables which relieves constipation and acts as an ideal "mucus broom" in the intestines. I do not believe that the human body assimilates "food-value vegetables" such as cauliflower, asparagus, turnips, potatoes, or from uncooked cereals. After a certain beneficial mechanical cleansing of the bowels through these raw foods, the one-sided raw-food eater lacks, in fact, the most important food substance, and that is grape or fruit sugar, unless they eat sufficient fruits.[62]

Significant and instructive is this experiment: Put a lemon in a moderate dry heat a few minutes, and it becomes sweet—like an orange. You develop grape sugar, but let it bake a little too long, or if cooked, it becomes bitter. On the same principle, all vegetables when baked improve by developing the more or less starch they contain into grape-sugar. This is true of carrots, beets, turnips, cauliflower, etc.

Raw fruits, and if desired, raw green-leafy vegetables, form the ideal food for humans. That is the mucusless diet. But the mucusless diet as a healing system uses raw, rough vegetables for their cleansing qualities; baked ones as food; and baked and stewed fruits AS A LESS AGGRESSIVE DISSOLVER of poisons and mucus to MODERATE THE ELIMINATION IN SEVERE CASES. That is one of the most important principles of the system, a point the raw-food fanatic ignores entirely. Eating raw potatoes, raw cereals, and unfired pies, is, in my opinion, absurd and worse than if they are carefully baked, which means developing the starch into at least partly digestible gluten and grape sugar.

Fletcherism

The American Horace Fletcher developed a complete dietetic healing system in itself, with great success on himself and others. His theory was to eat whatever kind of food you desired, but chew every bite 10 to 15 minutes. You may eat one sandwich a day and get rid of your trouble. The secret is simply this: It is a camouflaged fast; the stomach and intestines have a rest, the same as when fasting, and elimination is promoted, and the vital organs recuperate. But when continued longer, the bowels constipate from a lack of solid food and it is said that Fletcher himself died through severe "trouble" in these organs.

Another camouflaged fast in its effect is the Salisbury cure. A small piece of beefsteak and a little toast, once a day, nothing else. Relieves, improves, but never heals perfectly.

Under the same classification is the milk diet, which puzzles even the most advanced experts of fasting and dietetics by its partial successes in many cases. The secret is this: If you replace three "square" meals a day consisting of at least three courses each, with a few quarts of milk (liquid), the obstructions in the human engine are much less (read Lesson V), you feel better, and the body partially eliminates, and in many cases relieves, your trouble. But all milk-dieting patients suffer sooner or later from terrible constipation because milk is a first-class, sticky mucus-former.

Schroth Cure

This so-called "dry cure," founded by one of the great pioneers of naturopathy, is in its effect also a camouflaged fast. Three days eating nothing other than dry bread, with NOTHING TO DRINK; the 4th day, unlimited drink of light wine and some food, combined with all-night wet packs. This causes a tremendous elimination, if you can stand the severity of this "horse cure." Schroth[63] had marvelous success and a world-wide reputation; but many who had gone through this quick help many times came to my sanitarium, and I found they had very weak hearts and lacked more or less the elastic efficiency of the tissues. Read Lesson V again and you will understand the reason at once. I use the same principles of this cure in an improved form in cases where there was no reaction with a drink fast or by the mucusless diet as follows: 2 or 3 days nothing but dried fruits followed by one day of juicy fruits and starchless vegetables produces a most efficient elimination, but is only advisable for relatively "strong" people.

There are hundreds of other dietetic cures on the "market," and every once in a while one of them becomes fashionable; from the long fast and "fruit fast" up to the so-called "scientifically prepared" mixtures of medical and non-medical dieticians. The average health-seeker thinks that there is some special food or special mixture to be eaten for their particular ailment, and he or she tries everything—but always in vain, as long as they do not know or understand that there is but one disease—inside dirt, waste, and obstructions, and that these obstructions must and can be eliminated only—and systematically only—by the opposite of disease-producing, mucus-forming foods, that is by

"THE MUCUSLESS DIET HEALING SYSTEM,"

A mucusless diet, consisting of fruits and herbs, meaning green-leaf vegetables considered "unfashionable" since the time of Moses, that great dietitian and faster. (See Genesis)

The more we learn about natural laws that rule and govern our health, the less we need fear the destructive onslaught of disease. Only through a mucus-free diet can we expect to eliminate the accumulation of waste and obstructions deposited in the body tissues during a lifetime of wrong eating. Give the body a clean bloodstream and it will function harmoniously as nature intended it should.

---

[60] Reverend Sylvester Graham (1794-1851) was a Presbyterian minister and dietary reformer in the United States. He advocated vegetarianism, temperance, and the control of sexual urges through a clean lifestyle. Today he is most known for inventing Graham bread and crackers.

Dr. Emmet Densmore (1837-1911) was a medical doctor, inventor, author, and strong advocate for a progressive fruit and vegetable diet. He authored several influential books on health, including *The Natural Food of Man: A Brief Statement of the Principal Arguments against the Use of Bread, Cereals, Pulses, and All Other Starch Foods* (1890), and *How Nature Cures: Comprising a New System of Hygiene* (1892). With his brother, he also invented the Densmore typewriter.

[61] "Raw-foods diet," or a raw-vegan diet, refers to the practice of consuming uncooked, unprocessed, plant-based, and often organic foods as

a large percentage of one's diet. In practice, some raw foodists find it acceptable to frequently use blenders, food processors, juicers, and dehydrators, although other practitioners view these as forms of processing and avoid them. Some will also periodically eat cooked foods or mucus-forming raw foods. The term "vegan" was coined by Donald Watson in 1944 to draw a distinction between a person who abstains from all animal products, including eggs, cheese, fish, etc., from vegetarians who avoid eating meat, but still consume certain animal products. Once all non-plant based items are eliminated, the mucusless diet becomes, by definition, vegan. Yet, many foods thought to be acceptable in veganism and raw foodism should be avoided, or systematically transitioned away from, when practicing the *Mucusless Diet Healing System*.

[62] Many people mistakenly believe that Ehret's work is inherently, or only, raw foodism or fruitarianism. Yet, as you can see, Ehret emphasizes moving away from mucus-forming foods above all else. Although the highest levels of the mucusless diet are raw, mucus-free foods, Ehret advocates using cooked mucusless foods, and even some mildly mucus-forming items, when necessary during the *Transition Diet*. Details about the Transition Diet will be discussed later in the book.

[63] Johann Schroth (1798-1856) was a pioneering Austrian naturopath and haulage contractor. At age 18, his knee was badly injured by a horse and he successfully treated the affliction using cold compresses. Initially, he met a monk who advised him to wash his stiff joint with wet cloths several times a day. But as Schroth became tired of the repetitious activity, he developed a method of "wearing" cold compresses for several hours before changing them. Ultimately, the stiffness went away. Now being aware of the effectiveness of the newfound method, he started using compresses for wounds, bruises, swellings, and stiffness of the joints for both humans and animals. He eventually earned a reputation as a healer of domestic animals and subsequently used his methods on injured humans. Around 1830, Schroth founded a health spa at Bad Lindewiese that gradually grew to prominence. He introduced the use of steam baths and full-body wraps as forms of naturopathic healing. After he had observed that sick animals refuse to eat, Schroth propagated the idea of a strict diet for humans that included a regimen of intermittent days of dry and liquid fasting. His methods were touted as a means of purification and detoxification of the entire body by seekers of natural healing.

Confusion in Dietetics—Part 3

Lesson XIII

After this severe critique of all important dietetics, I must admit that I do not deny that all of them have, and have done, considerable good towards the development of the dietetic solution of the food problem and healing of diseases by diet.

Reviewing the entire development during the past 25 years, this fact remains: With the progress of chemistry, medical experts arrived at the following conclusion, "We now know exactly all of the elements contained in the human body, and therefore know what must be eaten for upbuilding—for replacement of used-up cells and for producing vitality, efficiency, strength, and heat."

You were taught in former lessons why these "conclusions" are wrong, and have produced the "protein" fad and later the "mineral salt" fad, and now the very latest fashion, i.e., the "raw food" fad. Without knowledge of the "great unknown," their conclusions must be wrong. This great "unknown"—unknown to the chemical and medical experts—unknown to the average person and health-seeker—unknown to the layperson dietitian—unknown to the general dietetic systems now in vogue—and this "great unknown," "O" in my formula "V" equals "P" minus "O," is the waste, the mucus—acids and poisons, the

OBSTRUCTIONS or "O"

in the sick, and also in the average so-called "healthy" human body.

In other words: If human nourishment could ever be figured by mathematical and chemical formulas telling exactly what to eat, you will still be fooled by nature—just so long as any ideal food is mixed with, and put into, this waste of mucus and acids already in the human system through years of wrong living. Nature confuses *you*— so long as you fail to recognize her facts and her truths—but nature herself is not fooled. To the average layperson, raw food reacts more or less mysteriously—as long as it is mixed with your own mucus—as long as it stirs up mucus and its toxemias in the unclean diseased body and eliminates these poisons. All laymen and experts covering the entire dietetic movement up to the present time are puzzled, confused, ignorant, and still in complete darkness of the fact that, in general, the average person *first becomes worse*, sometimes developing boils and all kinds of sores— "troubles" from "indigestion" when they start what they believe to be a correct and best diet—living on a radical fruit, mucusless, or raw-food diet.[64]

"Tell me what to eat," wail the sick, "I want a daily menu for my special disease" (like a drug prescription), and they then consider that as all sufficient. When the elimination sets in, they say, "These foods don't agree with me," instead of recognizing that the transition diet has already started in a moderate way to dissolve and to eliminate the old waste in the body—with some disturbance, of course. You must make them realize the necessity of putting up with this temporary inconvenience, and consider themselves fortunate indeed to be able to continue with their daily work instead of undergoing an operation, which would mean months in a hospital. The foods agree with them, but they do not agree with the foods.

Now you may understand why the mucusless diet is a system in which every change in diet has certain duties to perform—as a diet of healing to be applied systematically according to the condition of the sick.

You will now understand why and in what manner I differ from all others. The *Mucusless Diet Healing System* is not a collection of different menus for every disease; it is not "made-up" combinations of valuable and nourishing foods—it is not like a medical prescription or a compilation of standard diets suitable for all diseases, but it is a system of dietetic changes and dietetic improvements—a system of dietetic elimination of disease matter, waste, mucus and poisons; a system of slowly changing and improving the diet as a diet of healing towards, and up to, the ideal and natural food of humans—FRUITS ONLY—or fruits and green-leaf vegetables—THE MUCUSLESS DIET.

It is therefore a personally supervised, and in every case different, modified, scientific, systematical, progressive method of "eating your way to health," combined, if found necessary, with short or longer fasts.

It is a healing process *which every sick person must* undergo if they want to be perfectly healed; it is an exclusive dietetic "curing and healing, rebuilding and regenerating process" based on the use of harmless and natural food for humankind, "coined" and set biologically by the Creator in Genesis—"FRUITS AND HERBS," OR "MUCUSLESS DIET." Nature will do her part if we but give her half a chance. Try it out for yourself and watch for the results.

---

[64] In general, the removal of physiological wastes and encumbrances is referred to as "elimination" by modern-day practitioners of the mucusless diet. In addition to the removal of physical waste from the body, the term may also be associated with the uncomfortable symptoms that may arise during a period of great healing.

The term "healing crisis" is a commonly used and related naturopathic term that refers to a period of intensive physical and emotional cleansing. Common symptoms include the expectoration of various colors of mucus from all orifices, fever, aches and pains, headaches, dizziness and vertigo, mood swings, diarrhea, vomiting, loss of appetite, depression or anxieties, heart palpitations, localized pain at the area of obstruction, etc.

Ragnar Berg's Table (Revisited)

Lesson XIV

You can now understand that the dietetic problem is not solved, as the average person imagines, through simply knowing which foods are best and the kind of foods the mucusless diet consists of. In the previous lesson, you were taught knowledge unknown to all others— what happens and what must happen in the human body if the sick person eats only the "best foods" or takes a long fast. Later, you will learn how this stirring up and eliminating of mucus by "good foods" and fasting can and must be controlled by yourself, the treating physician, or dietician.

You may now see of what little value and how injurious it may become for the average health-seeker to stuff their stomach daily with terrible mixtures of "good food," "raw food combinations" (in the belief that raw food alone will do it), without any plan or system—without any regard for the disease and their mental or physical condition.

In spite of my antipathy towards "faddists," I will submit a selection of tables prepared by one of the most advanced experts of physiological chemistry—Ragnar Berg, of the special laboratory for food research at Dr. Lahmann's sanitarium of Germany.

Editor's Note by Prof. Spira on the Berg Table: The original Ragnar Berg table can be problematic and quite confusing for first-time readers, and many modern-day mucusless diet practitioners have wanted to see new, revised editions of the book that omit this chapter or improve it in some way. Ultimately, the purpose of the Berg table was to show that Ehret was not alone in believing that acid-forming foods were injurious to the body. The problem is that many of the items in the original table that are actually very much acid- and mucus-forming are listed as acid-binding.

Ehret does try to explain that the tables should be taken with *a grain of salt*. In the material that precedes the Berg table in the original text, Ehret explains, "The majority of foods he [Berg] calls 'acid-forming' is what I call 'mucus-forming,' and what he calls 'acid-binding,' that is, non-acid food, is almost exactly what I call 'mucusless'." The key phrases are 'the majority' and 'almost exactly'. Then he explains, "The mere fact that some foods given in the list are 'acid-binding' does not necessarily mean that I endorse their use. This list is given as a comparison only and should be studied for what it is worth. Please understand that I am not endorsing Berg's theories."

Yet, most readers tend to assume that the table is meant to be a "mucusless vs. mucus-forming foods chart." The chapter is more of an attempt to illustrate his alkaline vs. acid-forming food theories using the work of his peers. Most of what Ehret has published stands the test of time. Yet, the writings that do not tend to do so represent his attempts to dialog with his contemporaries, of whom he is greatly more advanced.

For the purposes of this twenty-first century educational edition of the *Mucusless Diet*, I've taken a great editorial liberty to provide a clearly defined list of acid-forming (pus- and mucus-forming) and acid-binding (mucusless) foods, as I have come to know them. I have also added new categories for acid-forming stimulants that are not necessarily mucus-forming, but are still injurious to the body and should be avoided or transitioned away from. One of the most useful aspects of the Berg table was its list of fruits and vegetables. I've included almost all of the food items from the original list, along with many other items in common use today.

Keep in mind that this is not a list of "what foods I recommend" on the mucusless diet, but an objective list of mucus- or acid-forming vs. non-acid forming foods. I do not recommend all of the items that are technically mucus-free, and there are some mucus-forming items that may be an important part of your transition. Many of the starchy vegetables or fatty fruits in this list may be used while on the transition diet. I also include a section for vegetables that are all, or *relatively*, starchless. Although they may contain a little starch, some of them have been identified to be great vegetables to use during the transition. Also, later in the book, Ehret will explain how cooking some starchy vegetables "improves" their cleansing abilities. Some vegetables that are quite starchy when raw become relatively mucusless when slightly cooked. **Pus-forming** and **very mucus-forming** foods listed below are the ones that should really be avoided from the beginning, if possible. But **moderately** or **slightly mucus-forming** items may be used effectively during the transition. This is not an exhaustive list of foods, but the most common ones are addressed. Ultimately, Ehret's TRANSITION DIET will show you how to use less harmful mucus-forming foods to get away from the worst ones. All of these issues will be explored in forthcoming chapters.

PROF SPIRA'S LIST OF ACID-FORMING AND

ACID-BINDING (MUCUSLESS) FOODS

PUS-, MUCUS-, OR ACID-FORMING FOODS

Flesh (Pus-Forming)

Blood of animals

Eggs (all kinds)

Lard

Meat (Beef, Chicken, Horse, Dog, Mutton/Lamb, Turkey, Veal, Pork: Bacon, Ham, Sausage, Gammon, Chitterlings, Pig feet, Wild game: Bison, Buffalo, Ostrich, Rabbit, Venison, etc.)

Margarine (made with animal fat)

Fish (Pus-Forming)

Crustacean (Crab, Crawfish, Lobster, Shrimp)

Fish (all types)

Mollusks (Clams, Oysters, Mussels, Snails, etc.)

Roe (Caviar)

Salmon

Shellfish

Dairy Products (Pus-Forming)

Butter, cow

Buttermilk

Cheese (all kinds)

Cream

Crème fraîche

Kefir

Milk (all animals and kinds; raw organic; skim, 1 or 2 percent, etc.)

Yogurt

Cereals (Moderately Mucus-Forming)

Barley

Breads (all kinds; Barley, Black, Rye, White, Graham, Pumpernickel, Zwieback, etc.)

Cereal grains (all kinds; Maize, Farina, Kamut, Millet, Oats, Spelt, White or Brown Rice, Whole or Refined Wheat, etc.)

Cornmeal

Pastas

Pseudocereals (all kinds; Amaranth, Buckwheat, Chia, Cockscomb, Kañiwa, Quinoa, etc.)

Beans (Moderately Mucus-Forming)

Beans (all kinds and forms; Black Beans, Black-eyed peas, Fava Beans, Butter Beans, Cannellini Beans, Chickpeas/Garbanzo Beans, Edamame, Great Northern Beans, Italian Beans, Kidney Beans, Lentils, Lima Beans, Mung Beans, Navy Beans, Pinto Beans, Soy Beans, Split Peas, String (Green) Beans, White Beans, etc.)

Nuts and Seeds (Mildly Mucus-Forming)

Nuts (all kinds; Acorns, Almonds, Brazil Nuts, Cashews, Chestnuts, Hazelnuts, Peanuts, Pecans, Pistachios, Walnuts, etc.)

Seeds (all kinds; Sunflower, Pumpkin, Hemp, Sesame, etc.)

Processed Foods (Pus- and/or Very Mucus-Forming)

Dried convenience foods

Fast foods

Frozen convenience foods

Packaged convenience foods

Processed meat

Confectionaries, Candy, Sweets (Pus- and/or Very Mucus-Forming)

Baked goods (all kinds including pies, cakes, pastries, etc.)

Candy (all kinds; Bars, Caramels, Chocolate, Fudge, Jelly candies, Rock Candy, Taffy)

Gelatin (Jello)

Ice Cream (Dairy and Non-Dairy)

Marshmallow

Acidic, Fermented, or Distilled Drinks and Syrups (Acid-Forming Stimulants)

Agave Nectar (because it is too highly processed)

Alcoholic Beverages (all kinds; Ale, Beer, Brandy, Champagne, Hard Cider, Liqueur, Mead, Porter, Rum, Sake/Rice Wine, Gin, Herbal Wine, Lager, Fruit Wine, Vodka, Whisky, Tequila, etc.)

Cocoa

Coffee

Kombucha Tea

Soft Drink (Soda Pop)

Syrups (Brown Rice, Barley Malt, Chocolate, Corn, Molasses, Artificial Flavoring)

Tea (all kinds from the Theaceae family)

Vinegar (White, Apple Cider)

Fermented Foods and Sauces (Acid-Forming Stimulants)

Fish Sauce

Fermented Vegetables (all; Kimchi/Cabbage and other veggies, Olives

Pickles/Cucumbers, Sauerkraut/cabbage, etc.)

Miso

Sauces with Vinegar (Hot Sauce, Ketchup, Mustard, Mayonnaise, Relish, Tartar, Barbecue, Salad Dressings, Salsa, etc.)

Soy Sauce

Vegetarian- and Vegan-Processed Foods (Moderately Mucus-Forming)

Chips (Corn, Potato, Plantain, etc.)

Frozen Vegan Breakfast Foods (Waffles, etc.)

Hummus (Processed chickpeas)

Lab-grown Animal Tissue

Margarine

Nutritional Yeast

Pasta (egg-free)

Pasteurized 100 Percent Fruit Juice (potentially acid-forming)

Plant Milks (Grains, Nuts, Seeds, and Legumes including Soy, Rice, etc.)

Plant-based butters (Nuts, Seeds, and Legumes including Soy, Peanut, etc.)

Plant-based Creamers

Soy Lecithin (food additive)

Tempeh

Texturized Vegetable Protein ("mock" meats including soy, etc.)

Tofu

Vegan Baked Goods

Vegan Confections (all kinds; Chocolates, Ice Cream, etc.)

Vegan Cheese Substitutes

Vegan Mayonnaise

Vegan Whipped Cream

Yogurts (Plant-based)

Oils (Fatty and Mildly Mucus-Forming)

Oil (all kinds; Avocado, Chia Seed, Coconut, Corn, Cotton Seed, Flax Seed, Grape Seed, Hemp Seed, Nut, Olive, Palm, Peanut, Quinoa, Rapeseed (including Canola), Safflower, Soybean, etc.)

Salts and Spices (Stimulants and Potentially Acid-Forming)

Black Peppercorns

Cayenne Pepper

Chili Powder

Cream of Tarter

Curry Powder

Nutmeg

Paprika

Pepper

Salt (Celery, Crystal, Iodized, Sea)

Vanilla Extract

Starchy or Fatty Vegetables and Fruits (Slightly Mucus-Forming)

Artichoke

Avocados

Banana (unripe)

Carrots (raw)

Cassava

Cauliflower

Coconut Meat

Corn

Durian

Fungus (Mushrooms)

Green Peas

Olives

Parsnips

Plantains

Pumpkins

Raw or Baked White Potatoes

Raw Squashes (Winter, Acorn, Butternut, etc.)

Raw Sweet Potatoes

Rutabaga

Turnip

ACID-BINDING, NON-MUCUS-FORMING, OR MUCUSLESS (MUCUS-FREE) FOODS

Green-Leaf Vegetables (Mucusless)

Arugula

Bok Choi

Cabbage

Collard

Dandelion Leaf

Kale

Leafy Herbs (Basil, Parsley, Cilantro, Rosemary, Thyme, etc.)

Lettuce (Green, Red, Romaine, Boston Bibb, Iceberg)

Mustard

Spinach

Swiss chard

Turnip

Watercress

Raw Vegetables: Root, Stem, Fruit (All or Relatively Starchless and Mucusless)

Asparagus

Black Radish, with skin

Broccoli

Brussels Sprouts

Celery

Cucumbers

Dandelion

Dill

Endives

Green Onions

Horse Radish, with skin

Leeks

Onions

Peppers (Green, Red, Yellow, or Orange)

Red Beets

Rhubarb

Sea Vegetables

Sprouts (Alfalfa, Brassica, Green-Leaf, Radish)

Sugar Beets

Tomatoes

Young Radish

Zucchini

Baked Vegetables: Root, Stem, Fruit (All or Relatively Starchless and Mucusless)

Acorn Squash (baked)

Asparagus

Broccoli (steamed or baked)

Brussels Sprouts (steamed)

Butternut Squash (baked)

Carrots (steamed)

Cauliflower (steamed or baked)

Green Peas (steamed)

Peppers (Green, Red, Yellow, or Orange)

Pumpkins (steamed or baked)

Spaghetti Squash (baked)

Sweet Potato (baked)

Zucchini (steamed or baked)

Ripe Fruits (Mucusless)

Apples

Apricots

Banana

Black Cherries

Blackberries

Blood Orange

Cantaloupe

Cherries

Grapefruit

Grapes

Honeybell Tangelos

Honeydew

Lemons

Mandarin

Mangos

Nectarine

Oranges

Peaches

Pears

Pineapple

Plums

Pomegranates

Prunes

Raisins

Raspberries

Sour Cherries

Strawberries

Sweet Cherries

Tangerines

Watermelon

Dried or Baked Fruits (Mucusless)

Apples

Apricots

Bananas

Blueberries

Cherries

Cranberries

Currants

Currants, dried

Dates

Dates, dried

Figs

Figs, dried

Grapes/Raisins

Kiwi

Mango

Papaya

Peaches

Pears

Persimmon

Pineapple

Plums/Prunes

Strawberries

100 Percent Fruit Jellies, Syrups, and Honey

Coconut Water

Fruit Jellies (no sugar added)

Real Maple Syrup (100 percent, no preservatives)

Honey (bee)

Transition Diet

Lesson XV

In the preceding lessons, you were taught the foods that are best, as well as those that are bad, and which are the worst ones.[65] You know the exact reason why, and also what is going on in the system—what happens with good foods as well as with bad ones in the human body. You have learned that even the best foods, which have the highest, most vigorous healing properties, can become harmful, even dangerous in the beginning if not carefully used; that they become mixed with the filthy mucus and poisons that they loosen up in the body, and thereby become poisoned, entering the bloodstream in this poisoned condition.

Everything is perfectly performed by Nature through evolutional, progressive changes, developments, and accomplishments and not by catastrophes. *Nothing is more incorrect* than the mistaken idea that a decades-old chronic disease can be healed *through a very long fast*, or a radically extended, strict fruit diet. "Nature's mills grind slow but sure."

My experience of over 20 years, covering for the most part the extremely severe cases of all kinds of diseases, has proven that a carefully selected and progressively changing TRANSITION DIET is the best and surest way for every patient to start a cure, especially for the average mixed eater. As long as wrong foods (foods of

111

civilization) are partly used, I call it a MUCUS-LEAN DIET. Transition means the slow change from disease-producing foods to disease-healing foods, which I call the MUCUSLESS DIET.

The speed of elimination depends upon quantities and qualities of food and can therefore be controlled and regulated according to the condition of the patient. The worst and by far the unhealthiest habit is the HEAVY BREAKFAST. No solid food should be eaten in the early morning at all if you desire to secure the best results. It is permissible to take the drink that you are accustomed to, but nothing else. If you find this difficult to do in the beginning, you may drink again later on, so that your lunch is taken in the empty stomach. This is so very important that *a number of light diseases can be cured* by the so-called "NO BREAKFAST PLAN" alone. (This subject is more fully covered in Fasting Lessons 18, 19, 20, and 21.)

It is best that no more than two meals a day be eaten, even though the quantity you eat is as much as if three or even four meals were eaten. Later, when the stomach is cleaner, a small dish of fresh fruits when in season may be eaten for breakfast if desired. If possible, the first meal, lunch, should be eaten between 10:00 and 11:00 in the morning, and supper not sooner than 5:00 or 6:00 in the afternoon. Another very important rule when eating for health is SIMPLICITY; in other words do not mix too many kinds of food at one meal. Count the different number of items in the average meal of today and the total will startle you.

NEVER DRINK DURING A MEAL. If accustomed to a beverage with your meal, *wait a short while after you have eaten* before drinking. Soups should be avoided with meals, as the more liquid taken, the more difficult for proper digestion. If a warm drink is desired, for instance as a breakfast drink during the winter time, make a broth by cooking for a long time different kinds of vegetables, such as spinach, onions, carrots, cabbages, etc., and DRINK THE JUICE ONLY.[66]

Menus for the First 2 Weeks

LUNCH: A combination salad, consisting of raw grated carrots or coleslaw[67] or both, half and half, and two or three spoonfuls of a stewed or canned vegetable, such as green peas, string beans, or spinach. Add to this one of the following items (whatever is in season): cucumbers, tomatoes, green onions, lettuce, or other green leafy vegetables, celery, etc., but only a sufficient quantity for a flavoring.

You may make an oil dressing according to your taste if desired, using lemon juice instead of vinegar—for flavoring purposes only.[68] The rest of the meal should consist of one baked or stewed vegetable such as cauliflower, beets, parsnips, turnips, squash, etc. If you still feel as though you were hungry, you may eat a small-sized baked sweet potato or one slice of toasted bran or whole wheat bread.[69] Fats of any kind, including ordinary butter, are unnatural and therefore should not be eaten. However, should you crave fats, it is best to use peanut butter or some other nut butter on your bread.

During the winter months, canned vegetables may be used when green vegetables are not available.[70] Drink the juice separately in the morning and mix the green or string beans or spinach, etc., with the salad stock as described above of coleslaw or raw carrots. The object of this menu is to supply the "broom" to provide means for mechanically cleansing the digestive tract by quantities of raw, baked, and stewed starchless vegetables. This may be called "Ehret's Standard Combination Salad," the "intestinal broom" spoken of so frequently and so necessary for properly eliminating the stored-up poisons now being loosened during the body's housecleaning.

SUPPER: Mix (half and half) a stewed fruit such as apple sauce, stewed dried apricots, stewed dried peaches, or stewed prunes with some cottage cheese[71] or very ripe bananas, mashed, sweetened with brown sugar or honey to taste.

The bananas would be for a less "mucused," or less acid, stomach.

Menus for the Second 2 Weeks

LUNCH: First a baked apple, apple sauce, or other stewed dried fruit. After ten or fifteen minutes, a combination salad as suggested in first menu, and bran or whole wheat bread toasted if still hungry. Cow butter should be gradually avoided and replaced by a vegetable or nut butter during the transition. By allowing the cooked vegetables to soak on the salad for 10 or 15 minutes, it serves the purpose of a dressing.

SUPPER: A baked or stewed vegetable, as suggested in the first menu, followed with a vegetable salad made of lettuce and cucumber or raw celery or a little coleslaw.

Menus for the Third 2 Weeks

LUNCH: During the summer, this should be an exclusive fruit meal—one kind only. In winter, a sweet dried fruit, for example, prunes, figs, raisins, or dates eaten with apples or oranges; or the dried fruits can be chewed together with a very few nuts, and then followed by the fresh fruits. If in the beginning this fails to satisfy, wait for 10 or 15 minutes and then eat a few leaves of lettuce or a cold vegetable either cooked or raw, *but just a small quantity.*

SUPPER: A combination salad as suggested in the first menu, followed by a baked vegetable.

Menus for the Fourth 2 Weeks

LUNCH: Fruits as in previous menus.

SUPPER: First eat fruits, either baked or stewed, or fresh, followed a little later by a cold cooked vegetable, or better still a vegetable salad.

If you find that you are losing weight too rapidly, the elimination should be slowed down by eating bread or potatoes[72] after the vegetables. Should you feel an intense craving in the beginning for meat—a great desire returning which you cannot resist, then eat vegetables only on that day, and NO FRUITS.

A Dissolved Mystery

The reason doctors and even naturopaths in general, as well as the layperson, do not believe in a FRUIT diet or MUCUSLESS diet, is simply this: Whoever experiments *without experience* with this diet of healing, whether sick or well, loses their faith immediately, as soon as they experience a crisis and become what they believe to be "seriously ill;" that is to say, a day on which a great amount of dissolved waste, debris, mucus and other poisons are taken back into the circulation, a day of great elimination. This produces at the same time a strong, almost irresistible craving for wrong foods and, strange as it may seem, the patient most strongly craves for the wrong food which was once his or her favorite. This is explained by the fact that Nature is eliminating through the circulation the waste of these foods, and it is when they are in the circulation the craving and desire is naturally enough produced.

This then is why it is of extreme importance that every meal of a diet of healing and cleansing *must leave the body* as soon as possible. Being mixed with the loosened and dissolved poisons, they cause these "uncomfortable" conditions—a fact that has never before been perfectly understood or explained.

Certain foods prove more laxative under certain conditions. *Therefore, eat the foods that you have personally found to be the most laxative in your own body.* If you do not experience a regular bowel movement before retiring, always help with an enema, a laxative, or both.[73] A natural laxative that helps, which you will undoubtedly find very efficient, is eating a few dried prunes before the other fruits are taken.

A very good aid to elimination, which can be used during the transition diet period until the bowels are cleansed from the old sticky waste and until such time as the bowels act freely from the new diet, is a harmless herb vegetable compound, perfected by myself, and the most efficient intestinal broom and bowel regulator known.

Formula for Ehret's "Intestinal Broom"

Quantities are given in "parts" so that you can prepare any amount that you require.

Note: All "ground" ingredients should be about as coarse as loose tea, the "powdered" ones about as fine as powdered sugar.

These are all fairly common herbs and you should be able to purchase them either at your health-food store or from any herb shop.

6 parts ground SENNA LEAVES

3 parts ground BUCKTHORN BARK

1 part ground PSYLLIUM SEED HUSKS

1/10 part powdered SASSAFRAS ROOT BARK

1/2 part ground DARK ANISE SEED

1/10 part ground BUCHU LEAVES

1/2 part ground BLONDE PSYLLIUM SEED

1/8 part powdered IRISH MOSS

1/8 part granulated AGAR-AGAR

1/2 part ground DARK FENNEL SEED

Mix the first three ingredients thoroughly. Then, combine the remaining seven real well and add this to the mixture. If you have a blender, it makes an ideal mixer for preparing this herbal formula.

The "Intestinal Broom" is easy to use. Usually a small amount, about the quantity that fits on half a teaspoon or less, swallowed with a glassful of water, is sufficient for adults. It may be increased or decreased according to your own reaction.

Other uses are sprinkled over salads, or brewed as tea: a half teaspoon to a cup of boiling water, remove from the heat, and allow to steep for 10 or 15 minutes. It has a fascinating flavor.[74]

[65] Non-fat fruits and green leafy vegetables are the best foods. Plant-based starches, grains, and fats are mucus-forming, but some of them may be used moderately during the transition phases. Meat and dairy are the worst foods and should be avoided at all costs.

[66] It can be very helpful to use vegetable broth to extend a liquid fast. However, be mindful to not lose control and eat the cooked vegetables used to make the broth. Overcooked vegetables would not be the best foods with which to break any kind of fast.

[67] When Ehret mentions "coleslaw," he is referring to shredded cabbage without mayonnaise or dressing.

[68] Ehret is against vinegar, although he does not explicitly say so. Twice he mentions that "lemon juice" should be used instead of vinegar for dressings. Some people believe that vinegar or fermented foods become alkaline after eating. Yet, Ehret suggests that the only acidic foods that naturally become alkaline during digestion are raw, tree-ripened "acid fruits." Although vinegar does not leave behind mucus, it is certainly acid forming. It is also a common relapse trigger that causes a mucusless diet practitioner to crave worse mucus formers. Thus, it is best to avoid vinegar.

[69] Many mucusless diet practitioners are able to use wheat products during the transition with no major problems. But like lactose intolerance, people's ability to tolerate certain mucus-forming foods is beginning to wane. In recent years, more attention has been paid to the negative effects of wheat products, as more people are starting to experience negative physiological reactions toward them. If you are sensitive toward wheat gluten (mucus), then avoid using it. Find bread that is made from gluten-free grains such as quinoa or buckwheat. However, avoid gluten-free items that use rice flour, potato starch, or other excessively gluey items. It must be stressed that if any kind of bread is used during the transition, it be very well toasted to aid in elimination. It should also be 100 percent grain (sprouted is preferable), have as few ingredients as possible, toasted well, and eaten toward the end of your vegetable meal. Also, it is advantageous to not eat any toast in the vegetable meals that follow a fast, especially as you become more advanced. It is best that such meals be mucusless. Keep in mind that wheat-free mucus-forming items may have the same negative physiological effects as those with gluten. If this is the case, then these kinds of mucus-formers will need to be eliminated earlier in your transition.

117

[70] Ehret wrote the *Mucusless Diet* before the existence of modern-day supermarkets that offer a wide variety of fresh fruits and vegetables from around the world, year-round. When available, it is always better to use raw fruits and vegetables for your transitional meals. Frozen fruits and vegetables may also be used when there are few fresh vegetables. If no fresh produce is available, canned items can be used as Ehret specifies. If used, be sure to obtain cans that have no preservatives, sugar, or corn syrup.

[71] One surprising item that Ehret suggests people use in the early stages of the transition is cottage cheese. Although it is dairy and certainly mucus forming, it eliminates relatively better than other dairy products. Yogurt also falls into this small category of transitional dairy products. This may be something to explore if you are coming from a particularly bad diet. However, it is certainly not a requirement. If you do not crave or feel the need to use cottage cheese, it is advisable not to do so—and it is certainly not something to be eaten after you have been transitioning on the diet for an extended period of time.

[72] As a rule of thumb, it is advisable to transition to baked sweet potatoes as soon as possible.

[73] The word "enema" refers to the injection of liquid into the rectum through the anus for the purpose of cleansing and evacuating the bowels. Many practitioners of the mucusless diet regularly use enemas and view it as a form of general hygiene. Enemas, or "internal baths," will be discussed by Ehret in forthcoming lessons. The word "laxative" refers to a food that stimulates the evacuation of the bowels. It must be stressed that Ehret does not promote the use of unnatural laxative medications or store-bought saline enemas, such as a Fleet enemas. Many modern-day practitioners of the mucusless diet exclusively use lemon juice enemas. For detailed instructions about how to perform lemon juice enemas, see *Spira Speaks: Dialogs and Essays on the Mucusless Diet Healing System* by Prof. Spira.

[74] Ehret does not discuss the use of medicinal herbs in detail within the *Mucusless Diet* except in this section pertaining to his intestinal broom formula. In *The Definite Cure of Chronic Constipation*, after discussing the danger of unnatural laxatives, Ehret says this about his formula:

> Among numerous laxatives on the market, those of botanical origin are the least harmful. After many years of experience, I have prepared a "special mixture" of this kind. It has the advantage of

removing the old, solid feces, obstructions, and mucus from the intestines, without causing the usual diarrhea and constipation as an aftereffect. It is to be used in the beginning only, as an aid, and will not have to be used continually. As soon as the intestines are cleansed from the retained masses of feces and other obstructions, and the mucusless or mucus-lean diet is taken up, you will realize the truth of the previously stated facts (*The Definite Cure of Chronic Constipation*).

Overall, Ehret supports the use of rational ancillaries that aid cleansing, such as herbs, sunbathing, exercise, colon irrigation, breathing exercises, etc. The criterion is that they help the practitioner safely eliminate constitutional wastes and transition toward a mucus-free diet. It must be understood that these ancillaries do not perform the healing, but the body heals itself once cleansed of waste. It would not be advisable to rely too heavily, or develop a physical or mental dependency, on any particular ancillary, including medicinal herbs. With the proliferation of modern medicine, people have become all too accustomed to getting immediate gratification from popping pills, and herbs should never be thought about, or treated, in this manner. True healing is not a "quick fix" but a regeneration that comes from removing all waste from the body. Ehret also does not advocate the use of any kind of nutritional supplements, as he does not believe that the body can use unnatural, isolated chemicals that do not come from fresh fruits and vegetables. According to Ehret, the primary power of healing comes from a mucusless diet with periods of rational fasting, or as Hippocrates said, "Let food be thy medicine and medicine be thy food."

Transition Diet—Part 2

Lesson XVI

Special Transition Recipes

Being known as a "diet expert," I receive continual requests for a "diet book," or at least a collection of food combinations, mucusless recipes, and menus.

Many volumes have already been published by numerous dieticians, which are now on the market. They call them "scientific diets," but not one of them is in accord with Nature, such as exists in the animal kingdom, and which is SIMPLICITY, with absolutely *no mixtures* at all.

I must again remind you that cattle, for instance, when in the wilderness eat absolutely nothing else other than grass during their entire life. No animal when eating combines different foods at the same time or even drinks between mouthfuls of food, with the possible exception of domesticated animals changed into mixed eaters by civilized humans.

The ideal, and at the same time most natural, method of eating for humans is one kind of fresh fruit, in season, and you will soon notice after you have been living on the transition diet for a while, that you will feel more satisfied and in fact are better nourished with one kind of fruit, than with all kinds of scientific mixtures or prepared, made-up foods. This condition cannot of course take place until your body is perfectly clean.

During the transition diet, I use food combinations and mixtures prepared from cooked, steamed, or baked foods for technical reasons, to better perform the healing process intelligently, systematically, and under control.

Vegetables and Fruits

My experience has taught me that only raw celery, lettuce, carrots, and beets combine well with fruits. In general, it is best never to use more than three kinds with the same combination. Always use one kind as the prevailing "stock" or base.

For a bad, acid, or "mucused stomach," use menus consisting of more vegetables and very little fruits. For a stomach in better condition, or the average stomach, use more fruits and fewer vegetables.

The following is an example:

1. FOR A BAD STOMACH: Take as stock 2/3 grated or shredded raw carrots, or grated celery or grated beets may be used, although carrots are best. Add 1/3 of finely sliced very ripe bananas and a few raisins or sliced dried figs. No nuts or cereals. NEVER MIX NUTS WITH WET FRUITS.

2. FOR A BETTER STOMACH: Take as stock 2/3 sliced or grated apples, 1/3 shredded carrots (or celery or beets). To increase the efficiency of this combination in its aggressive, dissolving functions as a mucus and poison eliminator, add more raisins, sliced dried figs, honey, or a fruit jelly.

Fruit acid dissolves waste and forms gases; fruit sugar ferments in the waste and stirs it up, also forming gases. Both eliminate and for this reason it *can become harmful* if they work too intensively. It is therefore advisable to use raw vegetables as a "broom" more frequently. For this same reason, use stewed fruits in the beginning, or at least half and half. For example, half raw grated apples (with the skin) and half apple sauce sweetened with honey.

122

A "Square" Meal Substitute

Before a crisis, during or shortly after, or to satisfy a craving for wrong food especially rich in fat, you may take this once in a while. While it is too rich, it is much less harmful than a "square" meal and will be found to be very enjoyable:

Take some grated coconut, mixed or eaten together with apple sauce, stewed prunes, or sweetened apricots.

Very ripe bananas—or if unripe, then baked—will be found to satisfy when unusually "hungry."

Other kinds of grated nuts or nut butter may be served once in a while for this purpose, but are too rich in protein and will produce, if continually used, mucus and uric acid.[75]

Improved "Cooked" Vegetables

Only one kind of cooked vegetable should be used at one meal. It may be eaten either cold or warm, and mixed with green salads and raw vegetables.

If cabbage, carrots, turnips, beets, cauliflower, onions, etc., are slowly stewed in very little water, or best, if carefully baked, they become sweeter, which proves that the carbohydrates are developed into grape sugar, more or less, and the mineral salts are not destroyed and not extracted. This is in fact an improvement and not a waste.

In winter, canned foods may be used as a substitute for fresh ones. I differ from the raw food "fanatics," because the food value is not important in a diet of healing. It is of more importance that the patient should and shall enjoy his or her change of diet during the transition, until their tastes and conditions have improved.[76]

Special "Mucus-Eliminator" Recipes

1. Raisins and figs or nuts, masticated thoroughly with raw green onions *at the same time*. These must not be eaten separately, to secure best results.

2. Grated horseradish mixed with honey. After mixing, allow to stand to take off sharp taste. The honey is only used to make it more palatable. 2/3 horse-radish and 1/3 honey, or to suit the taste. The ordinary radish, especially the black radish, may

also be used the same way, or finely sliced and eaten alone as a salad. For consumptives who cough without spitting, give one spoonful every once in a while. There is a surprising amount of mineral salts in radishes, especially the black radish.

Recipe for a Special Dissolver of Hardened Mucus and Uric Acid

With the following recipe, I once healed a woman who, after 6 years of paralysis, became entirely normal when both fasting and the mucusless diet failed to affect a recovery. It cannot be taken into a mucus-filled stomach. The recipe follows: Take the juice and pulp of four lemons. Grate and peel one lemon and mix with the juice. Sweeten with honey, brown sugar, or fruit jelly to taste.[77] The object of the sweetening is to make the mixture less sour and bitter.

Dressings

This is really a question of personal taste. A good salad- or olive-oil with lemon juice to taste is simple and good. A spoonful of peanut butter or nut butter dissolved in water and a little lemon juice added is another simple recipe. Add finely sliced onions (green) if desired. Homemade mayonnaise[78] that uses lemon instead of vinegar is not especially harmful during the transition diet and can be used if you enjoy it. Tomatoes cooked into a sauce or a good canned tomato soup mixed with the dressing may help you enjoy the "transition diet."

Drinks

Even if the use of table salt is discontinued, you will sometimes be very thirsty during your transition diet, because your mucus, now back in the circulation, and the waste of decayed unnatural foods, eaten with salt during your former life, is very salty. When in the circulation, you will suffer from unnatural thirst. A light lemonade with a little honey or brown sugar will relieve the thirst much better than plain water. The juice of any of the acid or sub-acid fruits makes a good drink and the best is sweet apple cider, if not too sweet. Postum,[79] cereal coffee, or even light genuine coffee, if this was your customary drink, can be used during the transition period.[80]

Supplement to Transition Diet Menus and Combinations

The "standard menu" of the day in my sanitarium, besides special prescriptions for patients under personal treatment, was as follows:

A drink in the morning

LUNCH: One or two kinds of fruits

SUPPER: Vegetables, mucus-lean or mucusless[81]

This diet quickly brings the average person, not called sick, into better condition. Slight spells may be manifested in some manner or other, but an "old chronic" or severe disease, caused chiefly through a drug-poisoned body, must be treated by systematically and individually prescribed daily menus, continually changing same, "speeding up and slowing down," according to the patient's changing condition.

The *Mucusless Diet Healing System* is NOT propaganda like vegetarianism or the raw-food movement; it is a clinical THERAPY OF EATING that has to be studied and intelligently advised and prescribed personally, the same as is being done by all other methods of drugless healing and therapeutics.

This diet heals every disease if it is possible to be healed at all, because all disease-producing foods are finally eliminated from the diet menus, and the new ones loosen, stir up, remove and eliminate, clean, heal, and cure the body.

You build up a new, and for the first time in your life, a perfect, natural blood composition such as the one defined in Lesson 8. This new blood removes and eliminates finally and unfailingly every disease matter, even though your doctor failed to locate exactly where it was.

The function of healing, the "operation without the knife," the cleansing, eliminating process begins almost immediately and must of necessity be conducted, controlled, and supervised for weeks and even months to secure proper results. The knowledge contained in these lessons is sufficient to enable the student to properly supervise their own individual case.

125

The menus, combinations, mixtures, and recipes are therapeutic adjustments to enforce the self-healing of the body, called disease, and not to suppress or to stop it as is done with drugs.

The average patient expects the right diet to help him at once; therefore the great desire for curative menus and mixtures. Even most of the advanced doctors imagine that a few menus and combinations from one day to the other is all the knowledge necessary.

As yet, they don't know the truth that you have learned in the previous lessons that physiology and pathology are fundamentally wrong, that all present-day ideas about food and nourishment are entirely wrong and diametrically opposite to the truth. Therefore, they do not have the slightest idea what happens and what must happen in the human system, if for the first time in the patient's life the decades-old waste and poisons are stirred up and have to be eliminated through the circulation.

You must realize and perceive that you are starting on an entirely new and perfect revolution, regeneration, and rejuvenation of your body when you change your diet in this way, and it cannot be accomplished within a few days by simply eating some good menus and mixtures.

Mucus-lean Recipes

If a little starchy food is eaten after a meal, it can be called a MUCUS-LEAN DIET.[82] But these starchy foods can be made less harmful by destroying or neutralizing, more or less, the sticky properties of the pasty starch. The more the potato is baked, the better. Toast well done is best.

Raw cereals should be roasted first, whenever desired, and will be found to work as a good intestinal broom, although they contain stimulants. Rice is a great mucus-former because it makes the best paste, but it can be improved by soaking overnight in water (you will notice that the water becomes very sticky and slimy and of an awful odor). Pour off the water from the rice and either fry or bake it a little.

A Mucus-lean Bread Recipe

Mix a rough bran flour or whole wheat flour with raw grated carrots (half and half); add only as much white flour as necessary to keep the dough; add somewhat-grated apples and a handful of grated nuts; also if desired, some raisins. Bake very slowly and well. This is best eaten when 2- or 3-days old or well toasted.[83]

---

[75] Ehret points out here that eating too many nuts will eventually create uric acid in the body due to their rich fat content. This is one of several statements that clarify the "nut contradiction" spoken of earlier in the notes.

[76] This is one of the most misunderstood aspects of Ehret's work. He does not view "nutritional values" to be important. What is important is food's ability to leave the body without leaving behind a great deal of metabolic waste. From this perspective, even canned mucus-free foods would potentially be better than raw mucus-forming ones. To this day, few diet experts have been able to entirely abandon additive nutritional concepts and, as a result, fail to understand this crucial aspect of Ehret's transitional approach.

[77] The juice of fruit such as apples or grapes may also be used as a sweetening agent. You may also dilute the drink with distilled water to form "lemonade," although this will make the drink much less aggressive.

[78] It is advisable to not use mayonnaise that contains eggs or vinegar. Today, vegetarian, egg-free mayonnaise is available, although it is hard to find without vinegar. Overall, I've found that using a sugar-free, fresh tomato sauce during transition is a more sustainable and much cleaner condiment.

[79] Postum is a caffeine-free powdered roasted grain beverage often used as a coffee substitute created by Postum Cereal Company founder C. W. Post in 1895. Post was a student of John Harvey Kellogg, who believed caffeine to be unhealthy. The Postum Cereal Company eventually became General Foods, which was bought by Kraft Foods. Kraft discontinued making Postum in 2007 and sold its production rights to Eliza's Quest Food in 2013.

[80] It is advisable to transition off of coffee as soon as possible. It is a very addictive and an acidic stimulant. The cleaner your stomach becomes, the more irritating such drinks will get. Water, or freshly squeezed fruit or vegetable juice, is always the best and most satisfying beverages. Once you are in the habit of juicing, and you experience the great taste of real juice, it will be hard to go back to coffee-like stimulants.

[81] This may be used as an overall rule of thumb for the transition diet. Sustaining this menu for extended periods of time is a good short- or long-term goal.

[82] The word "mucus-lean" refers to the period of dietary transition in the mucusless diet when mucus-forming foods are used along with mucusless ones. Mucus-lean menus are generally less harmful than standard mucus-forming eating habits by non-practitioners, and are an important part of the overall transition and systematic healing methods employed in the *Mucusless Diet Healing System*.

[83] Today, many 100 percent grain breads can be bought in the store. They are usually found in the health food or "organic foods" section, often in the freezer. Always look at the ingredients and avoid loaves with unrecognizable ingredients. In general, the fewer the ingredients on the label, the better it is.

Transition Diet—Part 3

Lesson XVII

(Vegetarian Recipes Revisited)

Some Improved Recipes of Salad Dressings

Condiments are much less harmful than mucus-forming foods. The so-called poisonous table salt is a very good mucus dissolver. The average mixed-starch eater could not stand this diet without salt.[84] Of course, with the perfect mucusless diet, the want and need of salt will be eliminated automatically, and with that, the unnatural thirst.

FRENCH DRESSING: Ingredients: 1 teaspoonful lemon juice, four tablespoons oil, 1/4 teaspoon honey, 1/4 teaspoon salt, and 1/4 teaspoon paprika. Mix 1-1/4 tablespoons of oil with the dry ingredients; stir well. Add the honey and the lemon juice. As dressing thickens through stirring, add the rest of the oil and a little garlic for flavor if you like.

Some Standard Mucusless Cooked Recipes[85]

As I said before, you may call the Coleslaw and Carrot Combination the "Standard Transition Salad." Now I will give you the Standard Cooked Mixture.

129

Serbian Vegetable Goulash

Stew, in a very little water or in olive oil or in a vegetable fat, coarsely sliced white or red cabbage and some sliced onions with some sliced sweet peppers, when in season, and finish stewing with some sliced tomatoes; a little salt and pepper if desired.[86]

Red or white cabbage with onions baked or broiled in a little fat and tomato sauce as a gravy is an appetizing dish. The same can be done with cauliflower, carrots, brussels sprouts, beets with the leaves, etc.

The idea is to bake as dry as possible and to afford occasionally an enjoyable harmless substitute for the chops, roasts, etc., which you have discontinued.

Some Special Suggestions Concerning My "Cookbook"

You will note that all menus and recipes are surprisingly short. If you fall back into the same gluttony-like mixtures, eating foods as described in vegetarian cookbooks and even in raw food books, you will never be perfectly healed. The ideal menu for humans is the "mono-diet," consisting of one kind of fruit in season and I must again remind you that no animal in freedom is a "mixed eater" at one meal.

You learned that I use partly cooked food during the transition diet and in the beginning the vegetables prevail. This has for its purpose the *slowing down of the elimination,* for it is well known that people *can stand* a stewed or baked fruit whereas they *cannot stand* the same kind when fresh. *Vital food* is not the entire object to be gained at first, but rather their property to dissolve and to eliminate. This vital healing efficiency is most perfect in all kinds of fresh fruits and will be found to be too aggressive for the majority of patients. This is undoubtedly the cause of the wrong ideas and reason for the "fruit fast" being in ill repute and it is the same reason *why I use stewed and baked fruits in the beginning to slow down the elimination.*

Whenever you feel bad, the cause is that you have too much dissolved mucus and probably old drugs in the circulation; then slow down the elimination by not eating raw fruits or even cooked fruits at all and for a few days eat cooked or raw vegetables only. *Vegetables work more mechanically and dissolve less.*

130

Later on, when the roughest waste is eliminated from your body and it becomes necessary, like in all cases of a severe chronic disease, to carry the elimination by the new blood deeper and deeper into the tissue system, the diet must be restricted more and more, as the healing process continues.

In the following lessons you will learn how a Fruit Fast must be undertaken, what Scientific Therapeutic Fasting is, and last but not least how the mucusless diet is properly combined with fasting if found necessary, or the principles and details of the *Mucusless Diet Healing System*.

Note by Fred Hirsch.[87] Professor Ehret frequently refers to having purposely omitted recipes, in spite of repeated requests, and gave as his reason:

> In Nature, such as exists in the animal kingdom, there are absolutely no mixtures at all. The ideal and most natural method of eating is the mono-diet. One kind of fresh fruit, when in season, should constitute a meal, and you will find yourself better nourished. This condition, of course, cannot take place until you have thoroughly cleansed your body of toxemic poisons, mucus, or call it foreign substances.

We feel sure that Professor Ehret would have approved and granted permission to include a few mucus-lean recipes, particularly of salads, in this edition of his *Mucusless Diet Healing System*, after being convinced as we have been that the public demand requires substitutes from the present-day acknowledged method of food preparation if they are to successfully take up the Ehret method. And so, with this thought in view, and with the hopes of converting many more to the Ehret System, we present a few tested recipes; successfully used at Health Cafeterias, where the tasty, delicious cooked combinations prove an agreeable surprise to the skeptic.

Numerous other equally tasty menus can be arranged by simply changing either the cooked vegetable or combination of raw vegetables.

131

The ideal diet for humans is the mono-diet and mixtures are prone to lead to gluttony, so that this should be remembered when arranging the meal.

1. ALWAYS EAT FRUIT FIRST. The digestion of ripe fruits takes place within a normal stomach within a few minutes after eating. Wait 5 or 10 minutes before eating your vegetable course.

2. DO NOT DRINK LIQUIDS OF ANY KIND WITH THE MEAL. Liquids of all kinds (including soups) interfere with proper digestion of the meal. At least thirty minutes should elapse before drinking both before and after eating.

3. HUMAN'S FOOD IS FRUITS AND HERBS (Genesis 1.29). For healing purposes, uncooked, starchless green leafy vegetables (parsley, carrots, celery, lettuce), combined with fruits both in their natural and cooked state, they will find to be much better than an exclusive fruit diet.

4. MIX BUT FEW VARIETIES. Fruit meals should consist of not more than two kinds of fruits in season. Your appetite will dictate the quantity to be eaten.

5. NEVER EAT NUTS WITH JUICY FRUITS. When nuts are eaten with fruits such as oranges, apples, pears, etc., the water makes nuts indigestible. Dried fruits, figs, raisins, dates, prunes, can be eaten dry with nuts. Chew together and masticate thoroughly. The fruit sugar helps to digest the nuts.

6. NATURE'S OWN BOOK IS SIMPLICITY. The fewer food mixtures the better. Three different varieties should be sufficient—four and five is often too many.

7. DO NOT OVEREAT. Mother Nature requires moderation in all things.

The following menus are simply given as examples of how to combine and prepare a meal:

Sample Menus

Cottage Cheese and Applesauce mixture. Add raisins if desired. Place on bed of Lettuce and serve.[88]

> A ten minute intermission between the fruit and salad courses may afford the family an opportunity of talking over the PLEASANT happenings of the day. And always bear in mind that laughter aids digestion.

Salad–Natural Vegetable Combination Salad

Baked Cauliflower: Boil cauliflower until about half done, and then bake in oven until brown. Use a suitable vegetable shortening when baking in preference to butter fat. Serve either hot or cold, and add dressing to suit.

Two pieces whole wheat or grain toast

Dried Fruit (such as raisins, dates, and figs) and Walnuts or Pecans (chewed together)

Salad–Cooked Combination Salad served on lettuce leaves

Baked sweet potato

Fresh fruit in season, such as peaches, apricots, grapes, etc.

Russian Salad (tomatoes, carrots, celery, watercress, onions)

Whole grain toast

Carrot and Raisin Salad

Ehret's Serbian Goulash

Whole grain toast

Applesauce with raisins

Coleslaw Salad: Finely slice raw cabbage. Add lemon juice to
soften, and allow to stand at least one hour before serving. Add
chopped onions, celery, and cold cooked carrots or peas. Add
dressing to taste.

Baked sweet potato

Mashed ripe bananas with fresh strawberries, and honey to
sweeten

Mexican Coleslaw

Baked banana squash

Cottage cheese and apricot jam

Lettuce and Tomato Salad with ripe olives

One cooked vegetable, such as baked squash

Baked sweet potato

Baked apple with honey

Elimination Salad

Baked artichoke.

Whole grain toast

Baked apple or applesauce

Baked beet tops

Whole grain toast

Salad Recipes

Natural Combination Salad: Mix a large bowl of finely cut lettuce; 4 handfuls finely cut radishes; 4 handfuls chopped tomatoes; and 2 handfuls very finely cut parsley. Add oil and lemon juice, mix thoroughly; let stand 15 minutes. Serve with dressing or tomato sauce, if desired.

May Salad: Large bowl of chopped cabbage; 1 cup finely cut radishes; 1/2 cup finely chopped sweet green peppers; 1-1/2 cups chopped tomatoes; 1 cup finely chopped green onions; 1/2 cup finely chopped parsley; and 1 cup chopped cucumbers (if in season). Mix thoroughly. Add 2 tablespoons lemon juice; 3 tablespoons tomato sauce as a dressing. Garnish with olives or radishes for decoration.

Apple and Celery Salad: Mix thoroughly 2 cups cubed apples to which lemon juice has been added to keep from discoloring; 1 cup chopped celery; 1/4 cup finely chopped parsley; 1 handful seedless raisins; and 2 tablespoons fresh oil dressing. Serve on crisp lettuce leaves.

Cabbage Salad (delicious): Mix 2 cups shredded cabbage; 1 cup finely chopped green peppers; and 1 tart apple, cut into strips about 1 inch long. Salt to taste. Add 2 tablespoons lemon juice; soak 10 minutes. Add 2 tablespoons dressing. Mix thoroughly. Serve on crisp lettuce leaves, decorate with chopped pimiento.

Carrot and Raisin Salad: Soak 1/2 cup seedless raisins in water about 2 hours. Mix thoroughly with 2 cups coarsely shredded carrots and 1/2 cup finely chopped celery. Add 2 tablespoons of fresh dressing.

Cooked Combination Salad: Mix thoroughly 1 cup diced cooked carrots; 1 cup cooked peas; 1 cup chopped cooked string beans; and 1/2 cup finely chopped raw celery. Add dressing or tomato sauce to taste. Serve on crisp lettuce leaves.

Serbian Slaw: Mix 1 cup coarsely chopped celery; 1 cup finely sliced cabbage; 1/4 cup finely chopped onions; 1/4 cup minced olives; and 1 tablespoon chopped pimiento. Add oil and lemon juice.

Fruit Salad (served in Apple Shells): Select good-looking apples. Cut off the tops of the apples and remove the apple meat.

135

Chop together equal parts apple hearts, pineapple, grapefruit, and cherries. Add lemon juice. Sprinkle with grated coconut.

Mexican Coleslaw: Mix 2 cups finely sliced red cabbage; 1/2 cup chopped celery; 1 cup red kidney beans; 1/4 cup chopped onions; and 1/4 cup chopped peppers. Add olive oil and lemon juice.

Carrot and Apple Salad: Mix 1 cup chopped carrots; 1 cup cubed apples, soaked in lemon juice; 1/2 cup chopped celery; 1/2 cup finely sliced dates; and finely chopped onions to flavor. Add olive oil and lemon juice; soak for 15 minutes. Serve on crisp lettuce leaves.

Summer Salad: Mix 1 cup chopped watercress; 1/2 cup chopped tomatoes; 1/2 cup diced cucumbers; and 1/2 cup diced celery. Add olive oil and lemon juice. Mix thoroughly and serve on crisp lettuce leaves.

Russian Salad: Mix 2 diced ripe tomatoes; 4 medium-size carrots, diced; 1/2 finely chopped onion; 2 sprigs chopped watercress; 2 stalks celery, cut in 1-inch lengths and split. Mix with dressing. Serve on bed of lettuce. Garnish with sliced tomatoes.

Asparagus Salad: Cook asparagus and cut into 3-inch lengths. Make a bed of finely sliced lettuce. Put asparagus on lettuce. Add dressing or tomato sauce if desired.

Cauliflower and Pea Salad: Cook cauliflower and break into small pieces. To 2 cups cauliflower, add I cup cooked peas and 1 cup chopped parsley. Add tomato sauce or other dressing and serve on lettuce leaves.

Asparagus and Cauliflower Salad: Boil asparagus and cut tips in 3-inch lengths. Boil cauliflower and break in small pieces. Mix together in equal portions. Add tomato sauce or other dressing. Serve on lettuce leaves.

Brazilian Salad: Mix 1-1/2 cups ripe strawberries, 1-1/2 cups cubed fresh pineapple, and 12 blanched thinly sliced Brazil nuts. Marinate in 4 tablespoons lemon juice. Arrange lettuce on plates in a rose shape. Fill the crown with above mixture; decorate with strawberries.

Date and Celery Salad: Chop equal parts dates and celery. Serve on lettuce.

Waldorf Salad: Mix well 1-1/2 cups diced crisp, tart apples; 1/2 cup lemon juice; and 1-1/4 cups diced celery. Drain off lemon juice. Add strawberry sauce. Serve on crisp lettuce; decorate with grated walnuts.

Mock Chicken Salad: Mix 2 cups finely sliced cabbage; 1 cup celery; 2 tablespoons finely chopped onion; 1/2 cup finely chopped green peppers; and 1 cup cooked kidney beans, cold. Add 2 tablespoons tomato sauce dressing. Mix thoroughly. Serve on crisp lettuce leaves; decorate with olives.

Grated Carrot and Spinach Salad: Add lemon juice to 1 cup chopped spinach and 1 cup coleslaw, and soak 10 minutes. Prepare salad plates with leaves of crisp lettuce, and arrange the bottom layer coleslaw, the second layer chopped spinach, and the top layer 1 cup grated carrots. Drizzle with one spoonful dressing and garnish with a ripe olive in the center.

Elimination Salad: Mix thoroughly 2 cups chopped spinach, 2 cups coleslaw, 1 cup fresh green peas, and 1 cup chopped celery. Add lemon juice and oil. Serve as desired.

Watercress Salad: Serve chopped watercress and 2 sliced tomatoes on a bed of lettuce.

Mixed Salad: Chop 1 large bowl lettuce leaves. Mix thoroughly with 2 cups chopped tomatoes, 1 cup chopped celery, 1 cup chopped onions, and 1/2 cup chopped parsley. Add lemon juice and oil.

Onion Salad: Mix 2 cups finely sliced cabbage, 1 cup sliced red onions, 1 cup chopped tomatoes, and 1/2 cup coarsely chopped parsley. Add 2 tablespoons oil and lemon dressing or tomato sauce and mix thoroughly. Serve on crisp lettuce leaves; decorate with radishes.

Cooked Vegetable Recipes

Stuffed Onions: Select six good-size onions. Remove a slice from the top of each onion and parboil until almost tender. Strain and remove centers to form six cups. Chop the cooked onion that was scooped out, and combine with soft breadcrumbs or chopped pepper and tomato pulp to create onion crumbs. Add seasoning to taste. Fill the onion cups with the mixture. Place in a pan and cover with onion crumbs. Add 1/2 cup (combined) oil and water. Bake until tender.

Spinach Loaf: Wash at least three pounds of spinach thoroughly. Cook in its own juice until tender. Drain and chop. Chill and add one finely chopped onion, and three finely cut celery stalks. Moisten with tomato sauce or other dressing. Mold and bake in pan 350 degrees F for 25-35 min. Serve hot or cold.

Spinach Cutlets: Wash fresh spinach and beet tops thoroughly. Cook separately in own juices until tender. Drain and chop. (Canned spinach can be used if desired.) Cook 1 cup fresh medium-size beets until tender, then dice. Braise 1 cup chopped celery, 1 large coarsely sliced onion, and one chopped bell pepper in cooking oil until golden brown. Place all ingredients in a chopping bowl and chop thoroughly. Mold into round patties or cutlets. Mix 1 cup coarsely chopped peanuts or walnuts and 1 cup whole wheat cracker crumbs or toasted whole wheat crumbs. Dip the patties or cutlets in the cracker crumb mixture and fry in cooking oil or olive oil. Serve either hot or cold.

Sautéed Sweet Potatoes and Carrots: Cook 2 cups diced sweet potatoes until tender. Cook 2 cups diced fresh carrots in a covered pot with as little water possible, until tender or use one 8 oz. can of carrots, drained. Combine the sweet potatoes and carrots, and sauté in a frying pan using vegetable or olive oil. Season to taste. Sprinkle with finely chopped parsley before serving.

Vegetarian Hash: 1/2 cup cooked lima beans, 1/2 cup cooked peas, 1/2 cup chopped celery, 1/2 cup toasted bread crumbs, 2 cups boiled or baked sweet potatoes diced, 1/2 cup diced beets cooked, 4 tablespoons cooking oil, 2 boiled onions chopped, 2 tablespoons whole wheat flour. Brown onions and flour in oil, add 2 cups hot water, cook until done. Add rest of ingredients and bake until brown.

Lima Beans and Cabbage Casserole: Cook 2 cups shredded cabbage and 1 pound package fresh-frozen lima beans or two 8 oz. cans (drained) in separate covered pots for about 12 minutes, or until tender, using as little water as possible. Alternate layers of vegetables in a baking dish oiled with vegetable oil. Dot with vegetable margarine; sprinkle with toasted bread crumbs and bake in moderate oven 15 to 20 minutes. Serves six.

New England Boiled Dinner: Cut 4 1/2 cups sweet potatoes, 1 cup carrots, and 1 cup turnips into 3/4-inch cubes. Slice 2 cups onions; Cut 2 cups cabbage into pieces about 1-1/2 inch square. Boil sweet potatoes and onions together. Cabbage may be either cooked separately or added to carrots and turnips when they are partially cooked. When all are done, mix together and serve with 100 percent grain toast.

Baked Artichokes: Boil until done. Remove from water. Spread open a few of the outside leaves and add garlic cloves. Place in pan. Pour olive oil over it and bake in oven at 425 degrees F for about 25 minutes.

Eggplant Hash: Cut an eggplant in half lengthwise. Place in oven until baked to a mushy pulp. Remove the peel. Mash. Add fried onion. Season to taste (tomato sauce optional).

Baked Beet Tops: Boil separately equal amounts of beet tops and spinach. Drain and chop. Braise onions. Add chopped celery. Mix all together. Put in pan. Cover with bread crumbs and bake.

Vegetable Chicken a la King: Mix 2 stalks celery, sliced; 2 cups chopped bell peppers; 1/4 cup pimiento; 1/2 cup green peas; and 1/2 cup cubed carrots. Add sliced onion. Make gravy out of tomato sauce. Serve on whole wheat toast or patties.

Mock Chicken Croquettes: Make a base of braised onions, bell peppers, and celery. Add mashed baked sweet potatoes, carrots, peas—or other cooked vegetables if preferred—and toasted bread crumbs. Mold and bake in olive oil until golden brown.

Vegetable Chop Suey: Braise coarsely chopped onions. Put in pan to sauté. Add chopped celery, bean sprouts, chopped bell peppers, water chestnuts, tomatoes to flavor. Sautee in oil until golden brown.

Vegetable Hamburger: Braise onions with bell peppers. Add garlic to taste. Cook together. Add toasted bread crumbs, celery, walnuts, and hominy. Mold and sauté in oiled pan. Serve with onions.

Baked Tomatoes: Cut (and retain) tops from tomatoes and scoop out pulp. Season pulp with grated onions and parsley. Stuff mixture into tomato shells and put tops back on; cover and bake at 400 degrees F for 25 minutes, basting with good salad oil. Arrange on bed of watercress or lettuce surrounded by sliced cooked beets. Use dressing desired.

Carrot Nut Loaf: Mix together 2 cups coarsely chopped carrots, 3 cups toasted crumbs, 1 cup chopped celery, 1 cup chopped walnuts, 1 cup mashed tomatoes, and 3 cups braised sliced onions. Add 2 tablespoons of melted vegetable or soy margarine. Place in loaf pan and bake at 350 degrees F for 1 hour.

Zucchini Italiano: Slice in about 1/2-inch thickness 2 good-sized zucchini and 1 good-sized tomato. Bake zucchini with 1/2 red onion, sliced; 1 small clove of garlic, if desired; and basil and oregano to taste for about 25 minutes at 400 degrees Fahrenheit. Add tomatoes and cook an additional 10 minutes or until tender.

New Sweet Potatoes and String Beans: Steam sweet potatoes and peel. Cook string beans with as little water as possible. Place both in a baking pan and add chopped parsley. Pour Italian olive oil over them and warm in oven for 15 minutes. Serve.

Vegetarian Corned Beef: Steam 1 cup each cubed carrots, coarsely chopped cabbage, sweet potatoes, and chopped celery. Fill a baking pan with brown gravy. Add steamed vegetables; brush lightly with vegetable margarine or olive oil, and bake 10 minutes at 400 degrees F.

Italian Meat Balls: Cook 2 cups whole wheat spaghetti in boiling water until tender. Meanwhile, mix 2 cups nut meatloaf, 1/2 cup onions, 1/2 cup chopped celery, 1/8 cup hot pepper (or to flavor) and Italian tomato sauce. Form into balls and fry in a pan at medium temperature. Serve with spaghetti and more Italian tomato sauce.

---

[84] Today, the degree to which salt is a dissolver and eliminator of mucus inside the body is a debatable point. As you eliminate the salt from your body, the mucus that you eliminate actually becomes much less salty. Overall, it is advisable to avoid table salt from the beginning. There are

many salt-free seasonings that can be found at stores, or make your own combinations. Garlic and onion granules can make a very nice seasoning. Oregano, thyme, and other herbs are also very nice to use. If salt is badly craved, sea vegetables such as kelp granules or dulse flakes make a safe alternative to iodized table, sea, or crystal salt.

[85] Similar to Lesson XIV with the problematic Ragnar Berg table, this chapter on vegetarian menus needed minor upgrades for the twenty-first century reader. First, it should be noted that much of this chapter was added by the book's editor Fred Hirsch, and not Arnold Ehret. Also, the menus in this chapter have considerably changed over the years. Items like protose (meat substitute made out of wheat gluten) that were heavily used in the fourth edition (1924) were eliminated by the 22nd edition (1994).

My goal is not to rewrite this chapter, but to improve on the menus presented. There are about five or six that I eliminated completely, as I find the ingredients or mixtures to be unsalvageable. Essentially, I eliminate all use of eggs (such as mayonnaise with egg, etc.), rice and milks. I also changed all use of white potatoes, which Ehret strongly advises against eating, to sweet potatoes which are almost mucusless when fully baked. And I got rid of most vegetaric meat substitutes and nut loaves, but left a couple of them for people who feel they need to use them in the beginning. Although some vegans may protest, I keep some of the cottage cheese combinations intact. Many people do not need to use such a menu, yet they can be very helpful in certain cases. It is not something that more advanced practitioners need to explore. Further, if you are transitioning properly, you will not be able to tolerate any kind of dairy for very long.

What I do not want to do is deprive someone of a transitional item that they may need or be able to use to overcome a challenging dietetic obstacle. Since transitional thinking is not finite, but ever-changing, the practitioner should know that such items cannot be eaten for extended periods. Those that only want to use the diet for a short period to heal will now have some things to fall back on that are better than a standard pus- and mucus-forming diet. Overall, for every bad item, there must be an item of lesser evil that is only a step away. Eating the baked banana, apple sauce, and chopped dates meal helped me get off of cottage cheese almost immediately. Wheat/grain toast, wheat spaghetti, etc., were all areas that I visited for varying periods of time to overcome hurdles. (For more details about how I used these foods in my own transition, check out my book *Spira Speaks: Dialogs and Essays on the Mucusless Diet Healing System*).

141

[86] Fresh vegetables should not be immersed and cooked in hot water, but lightly steamed or "stewed." From this perspective, "stewed" onions may also be viewed as "sautéed." An onion sauté is a great way to make the Standard Cooked Mixture taste great. To create a sauté, heat some olive or rapeseed oil in a pan and add chopped onions (and, optionally chopped garlic), and periodically move with a spatula until tender and slightly browned. Chopped celery and carrots may also make a nice addition to the sauté.

[87] This is an editorial note added by Ehret's original editor, most trusted student, and former owner of Ehret Literature Publishing Company, Fred S. Hirsch (1888-1979). This note suggests that many of the mucus-lean transitional recipes listed in the chapter were not put into the original *Mucusless Diet* by Ehret, but added later by Hirsch. There are also minor changes that have been made from edition to edition.

[88] Cottage cheese, applesauce, chopped dates, and a little brown sugar is a similar variation. Using baked banana instead of cottage cheese is a superior and much tastier upgrade to this recipe. To bake a banana, cut off the tips on both ends (leave the skin on). Place on a baking sheet and then into an oven preheated to 425 degrees F for 20 to 30 minutes. Depending on how ripe the banana was to start with, it may take a bit less or more time to bake. When it is done, warm banana juice will begin to leak from the two ends of the banana and the skin will be very dark. Take it out of the oven, make a slit lengthwise across the skin, and empty the warm banana meat and juice into a bowl. Then combine it with apple sauce and chopped dates. This baked banana menu may easily quench cravings for sweets such as cakes or pies, and is almost mucusless.

Fasting

Lesson XVIII

It is significant for our time of degeneration that fasting, by which I mean living without solid and liquid food, is still a problem as a healing factor for the average man or woman, as well as for the orthodox medical doctor. Even naturopathy required a few decades in its development to take up Nature's only universal and omnipotent "remedy" of healing. It is further significant that fasting is still considered as a "special" kind of cure, and due to some truly "marvelous" results here and there, it has quite recently become a world-wide fad. Some expert nature-cure advocators plan out general "prescriptions" of fasting, and how to break a fast regardless of your condition or the cause from which you are a sufferer.

On the other hand, fasting is so feared and misrepresented that the average person actually considers you a fool if you miss a few meals when sick, thinking you will starve to death, when in reality you are being cured. They fail to understand the difference between fasting and starvation. The medical doctor in general endorses and, in fact, teaches such foolish beliefs regarding Nature's only foundational law of all healing and "curing."

Whatever has been designed and formulated to eliminate the disease matters and designed as "natural treatments" without having at least some restriction or change in diet, or fasting, is a fundamental disregard of the truth concerning the cause of disease.

Have you ever thought what the lack of appetite means when sick? And those animals have no doctors, and no drug stores, and no sanitariums, and no machinery to heal them? Nature demonstrates and teaches by that example that there is only one disease and that one is caused through eating and, therefore, every disease whatsoever it may be named by humans, is and can be healed by one "remedy" only—by doing the direct opposite of the cause—by the compensation of the wrong—*i.e.*, reducing the quantity of food or fasting. The reason so many, and especially long fasting, cures have failed and continue to fail is due to the ignorance which still exists regarding what is going on in the body during a fast, an ignorance still existing even in the minds of naturopaths and fasting experts up to the present date.

I dare say there may not be another person in history that has studied, investigated, tested, and experimented on fasting as much as I did. There is no other expert at present, as far as I know, who conducted so many fasting cures on the most severe cases, as I did. I opened the first special sanitarium in the world for fasting, combined with the mucusless diet, and fasting is an essential part of the *Mucusless Diet Healing System*. I have likewise made four public scientific tests of fasting of 21, 24, 32, and 49 days, respectively, as a demonstration. The latter test is the world's record of a fast conducted under a *strict scientific supervision of government officials*.

You may therefore believe me when I teach something new and instructive about what actually happens in the body during a fast. You learned in Lesson V that the body must first be considered as a machine, a mechanism made of rubber-like material which has been overexpanded during its entire life through overeating. Therefore, the functioning of the organism is continually obstructed by an unnatural overpressure of the blood and on the tissues. As soon as you stop eating, this overpressure is rapidly relieved. The avenues of the circulation contract, the blood becomes more concentrated, and the superfluous water is eliminated. This goes on for the first few days and you may even feel fine; but then the obstructions of the circulation become greater because the diameter of the avenues becomes smaller and the blood must circulate through many parts of the body, especially in the tissues, at and around the symptom, against sticky mucus pressed out and dissolved from the inside walls; in other words, the bloodstream must overcome, dissolve, and carry with itself mucus and poisons for elimination through the kidneys.

When you fast, you eliminate first and at once the primary obstructions of wrong and too much eating. This results in your feeling relatively good, or possibly even better, than when eating, but, as previously explained, you bring new, secondary obstructions from your own waste in the circulation and you feel miserable. You and everyone else blame the lack of food. The next day you can notice with certainty mucus in the urine and when the quantity of waste taken in the circulation, is eliminated, you will undoubtedly feel fine, even stronger than ever before. So it is a well-known fact that a faster can feel better and is actually stronger on the 20th day than on the 5th or 6th day, certainly a *tremendous* proof that *vitality does not depend primarily* on food, but rather from an unobstructed circulation (see Lesson V). The smaller the amount of "O" (obstruction), the greater "P" (air pressure), and therefore "V" (vitality).

Through the above enlightening explanation you see that fasting is first, a negative proposition to relieve the body from direct obstructions of solid, most unnatural foods; second, that it is a mechanical process of elimination by contracting tissues pressing out mucus, causing friction and obstruction in the most circulation. The following are examples of vitality from "P,"

Power, air pressure alone: One of my first fasters, a relatively healthy vegetarian, walked 45 miles in the mountains on his 24th fasting day.

A friend, 15 years younger, and I walked 56 HOURS CONTINUALLY after a 10-day fast.

A German physician, a specialist in fasting-cures, published a pamphlet entitled, "Fasting, the Increase of Vitality." He learned the same fact that I did, but he does not know why and how, and vitality therefore remained mysterious for him.

145

If you drink only water during a fast, the human mechanism cleanses itself, the same as though you would press out a dirty watery sponge, but the dirt in this instance is sticky mucus, and in many cases pus and drugs, which must pass through the circulation until it is so thoroughly dissolved that it can pass through the fine structure of the "physiological sieve" called kidneys.

Fasting—Part 2

Lesson XIX

As long as the waste is in the circulation, you feel miserable during a fast; as soon as it is through the kidneys, you feel fine. Two or 3 days later and the same process repeats itself. It must now be clear to you why conditions change so often during a fast; it must now be clear to you why it is possible for you to feel unusually better and stronger on the 20th fast day than on the 5th, for instance.

But this entire cleansing work, through continued contracting of the tissues (becoming lean) must be done by and with the original old blood composition of the patient; and consequently a long fast, especially a too-long fast, may become in fact a crime if the sick organism is too greatly clogged up by waste. Fasters who died from too long a fast did not die from lack of food, but actually suffocated in and with their own waste. I made this statement years ago. More clearly expressed: the immediate cause of death is not a poverty of the blood in vital substances, but from too much obstruction. "O" (obstruction) becomes as great as or even greater than "P" (air pressure) and the body mechanism is at its "death point."

I gave all of my fasters lemonade with a trace of honey or brown sugar for loosening and thinning the mucus in the circulation.[89] Lemon juice and fruit acids of all kinds neutralize the stickiness of mucus and pus (acid paste cannot be used for sticking purposes).

147

If a patient has ever taken drugs over their entire life period—which are stored up in the body like the waste from food—their condition might easily become serious or even dangerous when these poisons enter the circulation, when they take their first fast. Palpitation of the heart, headaches, nervousness may set in, and especially insomnia. *I saw patients eliminate drugs they had taken as long as 40 years before.* Symptoms such as described above are blamed on the "fast" by everybody, and especially doctors.

How Long Should One Fast?

Nature answers this question in the animal kingdom with a certain cruelty, "fast until you are either healed or dead!" In my estimation 50 to 60 percent of the so-called "healthy" people of today and 80 to 90 percent of the seriously chronic sick would die from their latent diseases through a long fast.

How long one should fast cannot be definitely stated at all, in advance, even in cases where the condition of the patient is known. When and how to break the fast is determined by noting carefully *how conditions change during the fast*—you now understand that the fast should be *broken as soon as you notice that the obstructions are becoming too great* in the circulation, and the blood needs new vital substances to resist and neutralize the poisons.

Change your ideas regarding the claim "the longer you fast the better the cure." You may now readily understand why. Humans are the sickest animals on earth; no other animal has violated the laws of eating as much as humans; no other animal eats as wrongly as humans.

Here is the point where human intelligence can correctively assist in the self-healing process by the following adjustments which embrace the *Mucusless Diet Healing System*:

First—Prepare for an easier fast by a gradually changing diet towards a mucusless diet, and by laxatives and enemas.

Second—Change shorter fasts periodically with some eating days of cleansing mucus-poor and mucusless diet.

148

Third—Be particularly careful if the patient used much drugs; especially if a mercury or saltpeter, oxide of silver (taken for venereal diseases) have been used, in which case a long, slowly changing, preparative diet is advisable.

An "expert's" suggestion to fast until the tongue is clean caused many troubles with "fanatical" fasters, and I personally know of one death. You may be surprised when I tell you that I had to cure patients from the ill-effects of too long a fast. The reason will be clear later.

In spite of the above, every cure, and especially every cure of diet, should start with a 2- or 3-day fast. Every patient can do this without any harm, regardless of how seriously sick they may be. First a light laxative and then an enema daily, makes it easier as well as harmless.[90]

How to Break a Fast

The right food after a fast is as important and decisive for proper results as the fast itself. At the same time, it depends entirely upon the conditions of the patient, and very much upon the length of the fast. You may learn from the results of the two extreme cases, both of which ended fatally (not from the fast, but from the first wrong meal), just why this KNOWLEDGE *is so important.*

A one-sided meat eater, suffering from diabetes, broke his fast which lasted about a week by eating dates and died from the effects. A man of over 60 years of age fasted 28 days (too long); his first meal of vegetarian foods consisting mainly of boiled potatoes. A necessary operation showed that the potatoes were kept in the contracted intestines by thick sticky mucus so strong that a piece had to be cut off, and the patient died shortly after the operation.

In the first case, the terrible poisons loosened in the stomach of this one-sided meat eater during his fast, when mixed with the concentrated fruit sugar of the dates, caused at once so great a fermentation with carbonic acid gases and other poisons that the patient could not stand the shock. The correct advice would be: First a laxative, later raw and cooked starchless vegetables, a piece of rough bran bread toast. Sauerkraut is to be recommended in such

149

cases. No fruits should be eaten for a long time after the fast has been broken. The patient should have been prepared for the fast by a longer transition diet.

In the second case, the patient fasted entirely too long for a person of his age without proper preparation. Hot compresses on the abdomen and high enemas might have helped the elimination, together with a strong eliminative laxative and then starchless, mostly raw, vegetables; no fruits for a considerable time.

Through these two very instructive examples you may see how individually different the advice must be, and how wrong it is to make up general suggestions concerning how to break a fast.[91]

---

[89] To avoid using honey or brown sugar, you may add the fresh juice of several apples or a handful of grapes.

[90] Many modern-day practitioners of the *Mucusless Diet Healing System* perform regular lemon juice enemas. For detailed instructions on lemon juice enemas see my book *Spira Speaks: Dialogs and Essays on the Mucusless Diet Healing System*.

[91] Breaking a fast properly is of the utmost importance. I will reinforce Ehret's statements with the following rules:

Rule number 1—Do not break a fast with any mucus-forming foods. In fact, try to eat mucusless for several days after breaking the fast. You do not want to lose control if you start craving mucus-forming foods right after eating your first meal. You can either break your fast with a fruit meal or a vegetable meal. The fruit meal is more aggressive, and if you are not clean enough you could crave mucus afterward. A very laxative vegetable meal or salad can be beneficial. The key is to eat foods that create a laxative effect and travel through the intestines fast and efficiently.

Rule number 2—Do consistent enemas. In light of the above, one of the most important things during and immediately after a fast is regular colon irrigation. It is important that the newly loosened waste is kept moving.

Fasting may be viewed as an art form, and the ability to eloquently break one is the mark of a true master. This is one reason why short fasts are recommended in the beginning. As you gain experience with short-term fasting periods, you will learn how to maintain total control when you break a fast of any length.

Fasting—Part 3

Lesson XX

Important Rules to be Carefully Studied and Memorized

What can be said in general, and what I teach, is new and different from the average fasting experts, and is as follows:

1. The first meal and the menus for a few days after a fast must be of a laxative effect, and not of nourishing value as mostly all others think.

2. The sooner the first meal passes through the body, the more efficiently it carries out the loosened mucus and poisons of the intestines and the stomach.

3. If no good stool is experienced after two or three hours, help with natural laxatives and enemas. Whenever I fasted, I always experienced a good bowel movement at least one hour after eating, and at once felt fine. After breaking a long fast, I spent more time on the toilet than in bed the following night—and that was as it should be.

While sojourning in Italy many years ago, I drank about two quarts of fresh grape juice after a fast. At once, I experienced a watery diarrhea set in foaming mucus. Almost immediately after, I experienced a feeling of such unusual strength that I easily performed the knee-bending and arm-stretching exercise 352 times. This removal so thoroughly of obstructions, taking place after a fast of a few days, increased "P" —Vitality at once! You will have to experience a similar sensation to believe me, and then you will agree with my formula, "V" = "P"-"O," and you will realize the absurdity of making up scientific nourishing menus for health and efficiency.

4. The longer the fast, the more efficiently the bowels perform after it is over.

5. The best laxative foods after a fast are fresh sweet fruits. The best of all are cherries and grapes. Soaked or stewed prunes are good too. These fruits *must not be used after a meat eater's first fast*, but only for people who have lived for a certain time on mucusless or at least mucus-poor foods—the "transition diet."

6. In the average case, it is advisable to break the fast with raw and cooked starchless vegetables; stewed spinach has an especially good effect.

7. If the first meal foods do not cause any unpleasantness, you may eat as much as you can. Eating only a small quantity of food for the first 2 or 3 days without experiencing a bowel movement—owing to the small amount of food taken (another wrong advice given by "experts")—is dangerous.

8. If you are in the proper condition so that you can start eating with fruits, and you have no bowel movement after about an hour, then eat more or eat a vegetable meal as suggested above, eat until you bring out the waste accumulated during the fast with your stool, after eating the first meal.

Rules during the Fast

1. Clean the lower intestines as well as you can with enemas, at least every other day.

2. Before starting a longer fast, take a laxative occasionally and by all means the day before you start the fast.

3. If possible, *remain in the fresh air*, day and night.

4. Take a walk, exercise, or some other physical work *only when you feel strong enough to do it*; if tired and weak, rest and sleep as much as you can.

5. On days that you feel weak, and you will experience such days when the waste is in the circulation, you will find that your sleep is restless and disturbed, and you may experience bad dreams. This is caused through the poisons passing through the brain. Doubt, loss of faith, will arise in your mind; then take this lesson and read it over and over, as well as the other fasting chapters and especially Lesson V. Don't forget that you are parenthetically speaking, lying on nature's operating table; the most wonderful of all operations that could be performed; and without the use of a knife! If any extraordinary sensation occurs due to the drugs that are now in the circulation, *take an enema at once*, lie down, and if necessary break the fast, *but not with fruits*.

6. Whenever you arise after lying down, do it slowly, otherwise you may become dizzy. The latter condition is not serious, but you had better avoid it in this manner. It caused me considerable fear in the beginning, and I know a number of fasters and strict eaters who gave up when they experienced this sensation—lost their faith forever.

Fasting Drinks

The "fanatic" fasting enthusiast drinks only water. They think it best to avoid any trace of food whatsoever. I consider light lemonade with a little honey or brown sugar or a little fruit juice the best. Drink as often as you care to during the day, but in general not more than two or three quarts a day. The less you drink the more aggressive the fast works.[92]

As a change, vegetable juices made from cooked starchless vegetables are very good during a longer fast.[93] Raw tomato juice, etc., is also good. But if fruit juice—for example, orange juice, is used during a longer fast, be extremely careful because the fruit juices may cause the poisons to become loosened too rapidly without causing a bowel movement.[94] I know a number of such fruit or fruit-juice fasts which failed completely because all mucus and poisons, if loosened too fast and too much at one time, disturbs all organs too greatly

155

when in the circulation. This waste can only be eliminated through the circulation and without the aid of bowel movements.

Morning Fast Or Non-Breakfast Plan

The worst of all eating habits nowadays is to stuff the stomach with food early in the morning. In European countries, excepting England, no one takes a regular meal for breakfast; it is generally a drink of some kind with bread only.

The only time that humans do not eat for 10 to 12 hours is during the night while they are asleep. As soon as their stomach is free from food, the body starts the eliminating process of a fast; therefore, encumbered people awaken in the morning feeling miserable and usually have a heavily coated tongue. They have no appetite at all, yet they demand food, eat it, and feel better—WHY?

Another "Mystery "Revealed

This is one of the greatest problems I've solved, and is one that puzzles all "experts" who believe it is the food itself. As soon as you refill the stomach with food, THE ELIMINATION IS STOPPED and you feel better! I must say that this secret which I discovered is undoubtedly the explanation of why eating became a habit and is no longer what nature intended it to be, namely, a satisfaction, a compensation of Nature's need of food.

This habit of eating affecting all civilized humankind and now physiologically explained, involves and proves the saying I coined long ago: "Life is a tragedy of nutrition." The more waste humans accumulate, the more they must eat to stop the elimination. I had patients who had to eat several times during the night to be able to sleep again. In other words, they had to put food in the stomach to avoid the digestion of mucus and poisons accumulated there!

---

[92] It must be understood that Ehret does not have a strict or dogmatic definition of what is and is not fasting. In his book *Rational Fasting*, as well as the *Mucusless Diet Healing System*, Ehret discusses a spectrum of fasting experiences from water, to juice fasting, to all-fruit dieting. First he explains, "We need only to give a patient of any kind nothing but 'mucusless' food;

for instance, fruit or even nothing but water or lemonade; we then find that the entire digestive energy, freed for the first time, throws itself upon the mucus-matters, accumulated since childhood and frequently hardened, as well as on the 'pathologic beds' formed therefrom" (*Rational Fasting*). Ehret continues, "If you drink only water during a fast, the human mechanism cleanses itself, the same as though you would press out a dirty watery sponge, but the dirt in this instance is sticky mucus and in many cases pus and drugs, which must pass through the circulation until it is so thoroughly dissolved that it can pass through the fine structure of the 'physiological sieve' called kidneys" (*Rational Fasting* and Lesson XVIII, Fasting Part 1). Above, Ehret uses water fasting to illustrate principles related to the way in which the body cleanses itself. Here, Ehret highlights the notion that the body heals itself when properly cleansed of obstructions.

While talking about one of his own water fasts, he explains, "While sojourning in Italy many years ago, I drank about two quarts of fresh grape juice after a fast. At once, I experienced a watery diarrhea set in foaming mucus" (*Rational Fasting* and Lesson XX, Fasting Part 3). Since he had been water fasting, he viewed the fresh grape juice as breaking his fast. Also, Ehret's famous "public scientific tests of fastings of 21, 24, 32, and 49 days" (*Rational Fasting* and Lesson XVIII), conducted under strict scientific supervision of Swiss government officials, are water fasts. With that said, Ehret does not emphasize water fasting as the default modality for most of his own patients or advocate long water fasts. He explains, "As I have stated before, I am no longer in favor of long fasts. In fact, it may become criminal to let a patient fast for 30 or 40 days on water—contracting the avenues of circulation—which are continually filling up more and more with mucus, and by dangerous old drugs and poisons, and at the same time rotten blood from his old 'stock'—in fact, actually starving from necessary vital food elements. No one can stand a fast of that kind without disadvantage or without harming his or her vitality" (*Rational Fasting* and Lesson XXI, Fasting Part 4).

Ehret emphasizes the principle of transition and a GRADUAL CHANGE toward cleansing foods when he says, "If fasting is to be used at all, then start at first with the non-breakfast plan; then follow with the 24-hour fast for a while; then gradually increase up to 3-, 4- or 5-day fasts, eating between fasts for 1, 2, 3, or 4 days a mucusless diet, combined individually as an elimination adjustment, and at the same time supplying and rebuilding the body continually with and by the best elements contained in and found only in mucusless foods" (*Rational Fasting* and Lesson XXI, Fasting Part 4).

Ultimately, it is important to understand the various levels of fasting available to you. You will want to use the forms of dietary restriction that are rational for your physiological condition and experience level. Through Ehret's transitional ethos, fasting for humans in their current pathological conditions is a relative proposition. What may be fasting for my body may not be for yours. As Ehret implies, for some, just eating mucusless or a fruit-only diet could be a certain level of fasting. If you have questions or concerns about the type of fast that you should do, it may be advantageous to consult with a mucusless diet professional who can help you make the right fasting decisions.

[93] Be careful not to crave, and then uncontrollably eat, the cooked vegetables used to make the broth. You do not want to break a fast with overcooked vegetables, as they will not eliminate well.

[94] Also, remember that oranges and other citrus fruits that have not been ripened on the tree can sometimes be very acidic. If it is not possible to find tree-ripened citrus fruits, be sure that the ones you use are as sweet as possible.

Fasting—Part 4

Lesson XXI

You have just read in Lesson XX about patients eating several times during the night in order to sleep again. You have been taught why this happens. Upon awakening, you may perhaps feel fine; but instead of getting up, you remain in bed and fall asleep again, have a bad dream, and actually feel miserable upon awakening the second time. You can now understand the exact reason for this.

As soon as you get up and move around, walk, or exercise, the body is in an entirely different condition than during sleep. The elimination is slowed down; the energy is being used elsewhere.

If eating breakfast is eliminated from your daily menus, you will probably experience some harmless sensations such as headaches for the first 1 or 2 days. After that, you will feel much better and enjoy your luncheon better than ever. Hundreds of severe cases have been cured by the "non-breakfast-fast" alone, without important changes in diet, proving that the habit of a full breakfast meal is the worst of all, and most injurious.

It is advisable and really of great advantage to allow the patient to have the same drink for breakfast that they are accustomed to; if they crave coffee, let them continue to drink coffee, but *absolutely* no SOLID food! Later on, replace the coffee with a warm vegetable juice, and still later, change to fruit juice or lemonade. This change should be made gradually for the average mixed eater.[95]

The 24-Hour Fast, or One-Meal-a-Day Plan

As with the breakfast fast, you can heal more severe cases with the 24-hour fast, or in cases of deep chronic encumbrance and drugs, it is a careful, preliminary step to the necessary longer fasts. The best time to eat is in the afternoon, say, 3 or 4 o'clock P.M.

If the patient is on the mucusless or transition diet, let him eat the fruits first (fruits should always be eaten first), and after a lapse of 15 or 20 minutes, eat the vegetables; but all should be eaten within an hour so that it is, so to say, one meal.

Fasting When Used in Connection With the *Mucusless Diet Healing System*

As I have stated before, I am no longer in favor of long fasts. In fact, it may become criminal to let a patient fast for 30 or 40 days on water—contracting the avenues of circulation, which are continually filled up more and more with mucus and by dangerous old drugs and poisons, and at the same time rotten blood from their old "stock;" in fact, actually starving from necessary vital food elements. No one can stand a fast of that kind without disadvantage or without harming his or her vitality.

If fasting is to be used at all, then start at first with the non-breakfast plan; then follow with the 24-hour fast for a while; then gradually increase up to 3-, 4-, or 5-day fasts, eating between fasts for 1, 2, 3, or 4 days a mucusless diet, combined individually as an elimination adjustment, and at the same time supplying and rebuilding the body continually with and by the best elements contained in and found only in mucusless foods.

Through such an intermittent fast, the blood is gradually improved, regenerated, can more easily stand the poisons and waste, and is able at the same time to dissolve and eliminate "disease deposits" from the deepest tissues of the body; deposits that no doctor ever dreamed existed, and that no other method of healing has ever discovered or can ever remove.

160

This, then, is the *Mucusless Diet Healing System*, with 'fasting' as an essential part of it.

Fasting in Cases of Acute Disease

Hunger Cures—Wonder Cures was the title of the first fasting book I ever read. It gave the experiences of a country doctor, in which he said, "No feverish, acute disease must nor can end with death if Nature's instinctive command, to stop eating through lack of appetite, is followed."

It is insanity to give food to a pneumonia patient with a high fever, for instance. Having had an unusual contraction of the lung tissues by a "cold," the pressed-out mucus goes into the circulation and produces an unusual heat-fever. The human engine, already at the bursting point through heat, becomes more heated through partaking of solid food, meat broth, etc. (good, nourishing foods, so-called).

Air baths taken in the room, enemas, natural laxatives, and cool lemonade would save the lives of thousands of young men and women who are now daily permitted to die, the innocent victims of pneumonia or other acute diseases—due to the stubborn ignorance of doctors and so-called highly civilized people.

The Superior Fast

Please try and memorize the lesson on Metabolism (Lesson 6), because it is the most important truth of my new physiology. You should also memorize Lesson V and then you will clearly understand fasting with all its possible sensations.

All experts, excepting myself, believe that you live from your own flesh during a fast. You know now that what they call metabolism— "Metabolize your own flesh when you fast," is simply the elimination of waste.

The Indian "fakir," the greatest faster in the world today, is nothing but skin and bones. I learned that the cleaner you are, the easier it is to fast, and the longer you can stand it. In other words, in a body free from all waste and poisons, and when no solid foods are taken, the human body functions for the first time in its life without obstructions. The elasticity of the entire tissue system, and of the

161

internal organs, especially of the spongy lungs, work with an entirely different vibration. They become more efficient than ever before. They work by air alone and without the slightest obstruction. When stated differently, what this means is that "V" equals "P." And if you simply supply the "engine" with the necessary water that is used up, you ascend into a higher state of physical, mental, and spiritual condition. I call this the "Superior Fast."

If your blood "stock" is formed from eating the foods I teach, your brain will function in a manner that will surprise you. Your former life will take on the appearance of a dream, and for the first time in your existence, your consciousness will awaken to a real self-consciousness.

Your mind, your thinking, your ideals, your aspirations, and your philosophy will change fundamentally in such a way so as to beggar description.

Your soul will shout for joy and triumph over all misery of life, leaving it all behind you. For the first time, you will feel a vibration of vitality through your body (like a slight electric current) that shakes you delightfully.

You will learn and realize that fasting and superior fasting (and not volumes of psychology and philosophy) is the real and only key to a superior life, to the revelation of a superior world, and to the spiritual world.[96]

---

[95] This paragraph illustrates Ehret's transitional methodology very well. Here, he recommends a gradual change from a more dangerous substance, such as coffee, to improved substances, such as warm vegetable juice or fruit juice. Studying such passages can help you to adopt a transitional way of thinking that can greatly improve your practice of the mucusless diet.

[96] The nature of what Ehret describes as the "Superior Fast" is an interesting question. Above, Ehret says, "And if you simply supply the 'engine' with the necessary water that is used up, you ascend into a higher state of physical, mental, and spiritual condition. I call this the 'Superior Fast'." Some people interpret this to mean that water fasting is a "Superior Fast." In other words, that Ehret infers that water needs to be replenished through drinking. Yet, in Lesson V Ehret asserts that the body is an "air-gas

162

engine" that runs on air alone. Based on Ehret's arguments in this lesson, some interpret the "superior fast" to be what many people call a "dry fast," that is no substances other than air taken into the body (it must be understood that "dry fasting" is not advocated by Ehret and in most cases should not be performed by inexperienced practitioners or without supervision of a mucusless diet professional).

From this perspective, perhaps the H_2O created through the breathing process would suffice as the necessary "water" for the human body: $C_6H_{12}O_6 + 6O_2 \longrightarrow 6CO_2 + 6H_2O$. This equates to Glucose + Oxygen $\longrightarrow$ Carbon Dioxide + Water + Energy. In other words, oxygen coming into contact with the bloodstream produces carbon dioxide, WATER, and energy. As Ehret asserts, "The cleaner, the freer from obstructions, from waste, the body is, the easier and the longer you can fast with water and air alone!" (*MDHS*)

Ehret always makes careful distinction between the ideal "theory" and practical applications of fasting, and the mucusless diet. This often causes people to misinterpret Ehret's work, because the idealistic theory of fasting is seemingly different from the prescribed practical application. This also occurred when Ehret asserts that "humans are by nature fruit eaters" and that "the ideal menu for humans is the 'mono-diet', consisting of one kind of fruit in season." Yet, Ehret does not suggest that we can go from our current diets to an all-fruit diet overnight, as many readers have grievously misunderstood. Essentially, I find the "ideal" and "superior" theorized modalities for humans to be the destination that may one day be reached after the dedicated and effective practice of the *Mucusless Diet Healing System*.

Destructive Diet of Civilization and the Mucusless Diet, the Natural Food of Humans

Lesson XXII

You have now learned that total abstinence from food—FASTING—is the best and *most effective method of healing.* This proves with logical consequence how only a small quantity is in fact necessary to sustain life, and it justifies my oft-repeated statement, "The wonder is that we live *in spite* of our excessive eating, in spite of our eating such wrong, destructive foods." In the light of this truth, it almost appears ridiculous to note the endless fight and confusion regarding dietetics, protein, mineral salts, vitamins, etc. The potential food value is not the first question at all. You cannot heal drunkenness by water, without stopping the intake of alcohol. You cannot heal disease through any kind of adjustments, treatments, or diets without stopping the eating of the foods which produce disease, the latter being 90 percent of the present-day destructive diet of civilization.

I named the natural food of humans, fruits and starchless green leafy vegetables (as it is said in Genesis, "fruits and herbs"), mucusless diet, because mucus is the main and important and significant substance, while the other, wrong foods, contain, produce, and encumber the human body with the matter of disease.

165

The entire "trash" of scientific dietetics, food values, statistics, etc., is useless and in vain so long as the first step is not taken, and that is to see the foods and their value from a principally different angle:

1. How far and how much it produces and leaves disease matter (mucus) in the body.

2. Their dissolving, eliminating, healing properties.

For this purpose, I give you a special critique of the different foods, wrong foods especially, and you can see at once why they are "destructive" with no positive food value at all, but producing and leaving stored-up waste in the body. See Lesson XIV and you will find that Berg's investigations proved to be the same that I found by intuition, experimenting and through experience with myself and some thousands of patients.

Meats

All are in a decomposing state, producing cadaver poisons, uric acid in the body and mucus; fats are the worst, even butter is unusable for the human body. No animals eat fat.

Eggs

Eggs are even worse than meats. This is because not only do eggs have too high protein qualities, but they also contain a gluey property much worse than meat and are therefore very constipating, quite more so than meat. Hard-boiled eggs are less harmful, because the gluey qualities are destroyed. The white of eggs makes perfect glue.

Milk

Also makes good glue for painting. Cow's milk is too rich for adults and for babies, and it is plainly destructive. A baby's stomach cannot digest what a calf can. If milk must be used, then add at least half water and some milk sugar. Sour milk and buttermilk are less harmful and possess some laxative qualities; the gluey sticky properties disappear. Cottage cheese with stewed fruit (see Lesson XV) is good for transition diet. All other kinds of cheese are highly acidic and are mucus formers.

166

Fats

All fats are acid forming, even those of vegetable origin, and are not used by the body.[97] You will like, crave, and use them only as long as you can still see mucus in the "magic mirror." What doctors call heat calories is caused by the fats in friction, obstruction in the circulation; they constipate the small blood vessels.[98]

Cereals

Cereals and all flour products form mucus and acid. The worst of all is white flour, because it makes the best paste. Bran, graham, whole wheat, or rye bread are less harmful, because they have lost their sticky properties. When well done or toasted and well baked, they are much less harmful. Raw cereals, if toasted, are to some extent a mucus broom, but contain stimulants, wrongly believed to be "food value." Pies made of rough, unbaked dough, are, according to my belief, absurd. When eaten with sweets and acids, they are mucus and gas producers the same as French pastry.

Legumes

Lentils, dried beans, and dried peas are too rich in protein, the same as meat and eggs. The peanut is also a legume.

Potatoes

They are a little better than flour products, because they contain more mineral salts. They do not make a good, sticky paste. Sweet potatoes come close to natural sweets, but are too rich. Well fried or crusty, baked like Saratoga (potato) chips but without the animal grease, sweet potatoes are almost mucusless.

Rice

Is one of the greatest mucus formers and makes an excellent paste. I firmly believe through my experience with serious cases of sickness (awful boils, etc.) prevalent among one-sided rice eaters, that rice is the foundational cause of leprosy, that terrible pestilence.

Nuts

All nuts are too rich in protein and fat and should be eaten only in winter, and then too, only sparingly. Nuts should be chewed together with some dried sweet fruits or honey, never with juicy fruits, because water and fat do not mix.[99]

With the possible exception of nuts, the above represent about all of the foods which have to be prepared in some manner for eating; in fact they are tasteless unless specially prepared. What civilized people call good to eat, delicious taste, is absurd. If the tongue is clean from mucus, and the nose for the first time free from dirty filth, both then become in fact "magic mirrors," "revelation organs." We may call them the bridge of the sixth sense, that is, to sense the truth. You lose all desire for, and in fact cannot stand, these stimulating spices, especially table salt, any longer. All of these unnatural foods are extremely bitter, and in fact for a normal nose they possess an offensive odor. The sense organs of humans are in a pathological state embodied in "pus-like" mucus and waste the same as the entire system, and being in a partly decayed condition themselves, they find this half rotten food palatable.

Even then you would and could not eat fats or animal foods without the cook's "preparation," that is, the art to cover the real taste and odor by spices and dressings. In fact, taste and smell vibrations are so far changed from the normal natural, that the heavy meat eater does not like the wonderful odor of a ripe banana. They prefer "haut gout," a French word meaning "the smell of half-decayed meat."

No scientific food value tables will convince you of the truth. You must sense it with your cleansed organs, how wrongly you are fooled into believing that you nourish and build up health and efficiency by these foods which are in reality destructive, because they stimulate, or more truthfully, stop the elimination of your old waste until the day of reckoning comes, when you are "officially" sick.

Paradoxically, it is true that civilized people starve to death through ten times too much overeating of wrong, destructive foods. The "sack" (stomach) of digestion is enlarged and sunken, prolapsed, which condition dislocates and interferes with the proper functioning of the other organs. Its gland and pores of the walls are totally

168

constipated and its elasticity, as well as that of the intestines, with its vital function almost paralyzed. The abdomen is an abnormally enlarged sack of fatty, watery, dislocated organs through which half or even more of the decayed foods of civilization slide. It ferments more and more into feces such as no animal has, *and this is called digestion!*

Natural Food of Man is the title of a book by Hereward Carrington.[100]

There are some others by European authors who prove and show from every point of view that humans have, and must have, lived in prehistoric times from unfired, natural foods, fruits, and green-leaf vegetables; however, a great philosopher once said, "Whatever must be first proved is doubtful." Whoever does not see or sense the truth at once will never believe it, even if it is proven thousands of times and from every possible angle. Even experts of fruit diet and raw-food advocates have doubts that the degenerate humans of today can live the paradisiacal life.

It took me a few years of continual testing and experimenting until I was thoroughly convinced in spite of the fact that I believed at once. Now memorize what I teach in Lesson V and in the lessons on the new physiology. All others are on the wrong track, misled by the protein fad as well as through ignorance of how it looks inside of the body, what disease is, etc., but especially obstructive to recognition of the truth is the ignorance as to what happens in the body if you eat fruits, fast, or live on a mucusless diet. This fact that the interpretation of all and every sensation, which becomes more and more strange and new, the more and deeper healing process goes on, is based on the Old Physiology, and is therefore and must be consequently wrong. It is and was the "stumbling block" in the enlightenment about drugless healing in the first place, and advanced dietetics in particular. The natural diet was never systemically taken up, especially in combination with fasting, based on the truth of my new but correct physiology. This is absolutely necessary to learn and to understand. If you believe and know unshakably the truth of Lesson V, as well as the other lessons bearing on this subject, you will never doubt any more that fruits alone, even of but one kind, not only heal but nourish perfectly the human body, eliminating entirely the possibility of disease.

All others, not knowing these new truths and not possessing the necessary knowledge contained only in the *Mucusless Diet Healing System* can never secure a perfectly clean body and complete healing as well as possess an understanding of every situation.

They will never believe in the divine perfectness of the "Bread of Heaven," as it is said, "The Lord will punish them by blindness," spiritual blindness, meaning that doubt, losing faith and belief, will return again and again as long as waste and old poisons are circulating through the brain for elimination. You are saved from this tragic error, I hope.

The more free you become from any kind of waste and poisons, the more you will sense, feel, and believe this greatest of all truths: "That the Paradisiacal diet is not only sufficient but brings you higher and higher into physical and mental conditions never before experienced."

---

[97] As mentioned earlier, many readers assume that avocados are mucus-free because they are technically a "fruit." Although avocados are not addressed specifically by Ehret—as they did not become a prevalent salad item until the 1950s—Ehret clearly indicates that all fat-containing foods, including those of vegetable origin, are mucus-forming. Avocados have become a staple food for many self-identified raw-foodists, vegans, and fruitarians. From the perspective of the mucusless diet, it is important to be mindful of how much you eat fatty fruits, or avoid them completely. If they are being eaten, it is best to begin mindfully transitioning off them.

[98] Ehret does not say much about the calorie theory, which suggests his disregard for it. The term "calorie" (circa 1865) derives from the Latin calor, gen. caloris, meaning "heat." The large calorie, also called the dietary or nutritional calorie, is the amount of energy needed to raise the temperature of one kilogram of water by one degree Celsius. A calorimeter, invented by Wilbur Olin Atwater (1844-1907), is the device used to measure the heat of chemical reactions as well as heat capacity. What is known as "food energy" is defined as the amount of energy obtained from food available through cellular respiration. Based on the first law of thermodynamics, that energy can neither be created nor destroyed but only changed from one form to

170

another, Atwater theorized that the amount of unused food energy is left over and stored in the body. Atwater reported on the weight of the calorie as a means to measure the efficiency of a diet. He stated that different types of food produced different amounts of energy, and he advocated that the optimal diet should include mostly proteins, beans, and vegetables, while fats and fruits were to be avoided (see *Principles of Nutrition and Nutritive Value of Food* by Atwater, 1904).

But, how is it possible for a calorimeter to incinerate food like a human body does? It simply does not. The way in which the body metabolizes food does not resemble the burning process used in a calorimeter. The way in which calories are conceived of in the dietary realm has shifted a bit since Ehret's time, although fats are still estimated to represent nine calories per gram, carbohydrates and proteins four, and fiber (sometimes counted separately) two. Since Atwater's day, the practice of counting calories to restrict food intake in the hopes of losing weight has remained in fashion.

The concept of calories is, at best, not useful and outdated, while the fanaticism surrounding it is most unfortunate. Ultimately, counting calories, or the food energy, of fruit and vegetables in the same way as a bag of white potato chips or a steak is the height of folly. From Ehret's perspective, the latter two are not foodstuffs fit for humans. How many calories does bleach have? Since we do not consider it to be food, the calculation has not been made. Humans, as a tropical frugivorous species, survived for years without endeavoring to measure the amount of heat it takes to raise the temperature of 1 kilogram of water by 1 degree Celsius (1 "large" calorie). Such thinking has nurtured a fundamentally flawed notion of nutrition and metabolism, and enabled people to rationalize eating harmful substances. From Ehret's perspective, what Western dietitians view as "energy" from mucus-forming foods is nothing more than "stimulation" from a poison. Energy, i.e. true vitality in the human body, exists only in an internal environment that is free of acidic wastes, mucus, and uneliminated toxic foreign matters. For more on Ehret's theory of human vitality, see Lesson V.

[99] Earlier in the book, nuts are listed as mucusless. However, that contradicts what is said about nuts here. Ehret explains that all fats are mucus or acid forming. To be clear, nuts are mucus-forming foods. As mentioned earlier, they should always be eaten with dried fruits such as raisins to aid in digestion, and in moderation during the transition.

171

[100] Hereward Carrington, PhD. (1880-1958) was a well-known British author and investigator of psychic phenomena. His subjects included several of the most high-profile cases of apparent psychic ability of his time, and he wrote over 100 books on subjects including paranormal and psychical research, and progressive health. His most famous book, *The Natural Food of Man: A Brief Statement of the Principal Arguments against the use of Bread, Cereals, Pulses, and all other Starch Goods* (1912) explores the fruitarian nature of human-beings.

Lesson XXIII

Sex Diseases

Through the knowledge received in past lessons, you now know and can realize more than any naturopath that there is no principal difference between any one kind of disease or another.

In this particular case, however, we find an exception, but only in so far as the symptoms of syphilis are concerned. Venereal diseases can be healed by diet and fasting easily for the simple reason that the patient is generally young in years. The cure becomes more aggravated, made more difficult, if drugs have been used. This, of course, has unfortunately happened in almost every case.

The so-called, characteristic symptoms of any kind of syphilitic disease are due to drugs of one or several kinds.

Gonorrhea

Nothing is easier to heal than this "cold" or "catarrh" at the sex organ, if untouched by drugs or injections. Doctors must admit that this condition may exist *without actual sex intercourse*, and therefore the germ can hardly be blamed. Gonorrhea is simply an elimination through this natural elimination organ. One-sided meat eaters are very susceptible to this disease. Should a society girl contract it, they call it Leucorrhea.

If drug injections are used for any continued length of time, the mucus and pus are thrown back into the prostatic gland, bladder, etc. In case of the female, the entire womb—uterus—becomes inflamed, producing all kinds of typical woman diseases.

I had hundreds of such cases where naturopathy failed to heal. Only fasting and this diet can help.

Roseola or rose rash, a syphilitic eczema, characterized by its "ham-gray" shade, the gray shade of the whites of the eye, is due to saltpeter acid, silver oxide injections. This also is the cause if gonorrhea enters the bone. All three are called syphilitic symptoms. Mercury is to blame for the hard chancre, secondary, and tertiary syphilis.

The so-called "syphilis" does not exist in the animal kingdom or among uncivilized people. Drugs are to blame for these destructive diseases, together with the diet of civilization. Sexual excesses are, of course, also to be blamed, but knowing exactly what disease is, you may agree if I expose the "mystery" of this disease with one stroke, i.e., drugs and extreme meat diet of civilization are far more to blame than all sexual excesses together.

For a patient poisoned especially by mercury, a very careful and long transition diet is necessary.[101] A radical fruit diet or fast may become harmful, not through it, but caused by the drugs when they are dissolved and are back in the bloodstream for elimination.

This condition requires so careful a control of the elimination that under all circumstances an expert with previous experience is required.

The so-very-common disease of dislocation, or falling of the womb, can be healed, and only by this diet, together with long fastings combined with short fasts and with a long preparative diet.

I have saved hundreds of patients suffering from prostatic gland inflammation, stricture, bladder disease, from the tortures of doctors. I have facilitated cures even after naturopathy had failed by natural

174

methods of elimination through a new and perfect blood composition resulting from a mucusless diet.

Sex Psychology

It is significant for our civilization that sexual intercourse is seen as an immoral act. It is yet in the shade of a mystery. From a natural moral standpoint, says a philosopher, an unclean person has no right to produce a new being. "You shall not only generate, but reproduce yourself," says that great thinker, Nietzsche.

The fact is that we are all, with a very few exceptions, the cause of stimulants instead of love vibrations exclusively. Procreation is the most holy and divine act and charged with the highest responsibility, especially on the part of the father. A germ with the slightest defect is a generation not forward but backward. In ancient classical civilizations, "sex" was a cult, a religion, and in most mythological poetry of all civilized people, love is the great, main, and general subject with the conscious or unconscious goal to reproduce their kind.

The fact is proven by statistics that every family of the city's population dies out, disappears with the third or fourth generation. In other words, the "sins" of the fathers and of the mothers produce diseased children and children's children degenerating into death with the third generation. What are these "sins?" You shall "love thy neighbor," and you do, perhaps, but you kill your own child, partly at least before it is born. Latent disease is general and universal. How can a defective germ grow into a perfect being between a filthy, mostly constipated colon and an unclean bladder of a civilized mother? And one of the worst tragedies of ignorance is the expectant mother who eats twice as much decayed "cadavers" of animals killed years ago in the stock yards of Chicago, because she is advised to "*eat for two*"—herself and the growing embryo.

Natural Control of Sex

"Nothing above the truth!—Confess your sins to your own heart." It is a blasphemic paradox, tragic (there is no word strong enough) condition to stimulate a function continually with enforcement ignorantly expecting thereby to grow healthy and happy,

175

believing you can suppress or control this function by preaching morals.

Nature does not listen to you, but you must listen to Nature if you want to be happy. We are the product of stimulations, and not of natural love vibrations, which eventually leads to impotence.

The only way to heal impotence is through fasting and this diet. (See Lesson V) Sex is a part of vitality; it is even, so to say, the barometer of regeneration, rejuvenation, youth, health, and happiness.

I have seen sterility of the female healed, and every patient who earnestly took up this system for any kind of disease "rejuvenated."

No one of western civilization knows what genuine "love vibrations" mean from a body with clean blood composed of such ingredients that produce electric currents and static electricity sent out and received by "wireless"—hair. See what I have to say about hair in my *Rational Fasting*. The beard of man is a secondary sex organ. Beardless and hairless and bald makes for a "second-rate" sex quality in every respect. See Judges 16:13-18.[102]

If you could believe how easy it is to control sex by this diet, you would soon quit your steaks and eggs.

Masturbation, night emissions, prostitution, etc., are all eliminated from the sex life of anyone living on a mucusless diet after their body has become clean and powerful.

That saying, "keeping the germ (an idea of modern experts) will nourish a person's brain (high protein substance)" is absurd. Love is the greatest power and it is, if natural, the highest "invisible food" from the infinite for soul and body.

---

[101] For more on mercury, see note 28.

[102] In the Hebrew Bible, Samson (meaning "man of the sun") is granted supernatural strength by God in order to combat his enemies and perform heroic feats. His two fatal flaws, however, are his attraction to deceptive women and his hair, without the latter of which he would lose his power and vitality. In these verses, Delilah is trying to discover what gives Samson

his great strength so that she may find a way to subdue him. He finally admits that his hair had never been cut and that it is the source of his great strength (verses 13-20 are included to provide greater context):

> Judges 16:13-20 (New American Bible): So Delilah took new ropes and bound him with them and said to him, "The Philistines are upon you, Samson!" For the men were lying in wait in the inner room. But he snapped the ropes from his arms like a thread. Then Delilah said to Samson, "Up to now you have deceived me and told me lies; tell me how you may be bound." And he said to her, "If you weave the seven locks of my hair with the web and fasten it with a pin, then I will become weak and be like any other man." So while he slept, Delilah took the seven locks of his hair and wove them into the web. And she fastened it with the pin and said to him, "The Philistines are upon you, Samson!" But he awoke from his sleep and pulled out the pin of the loom and the web. Then she said to him, "How can you say that you love me when you do not confide in me? Three times already you have mocked me and not told me the secret of your great strength!" She importuned him continually and vexed him with her complaints till he was deathly weary of them. So he took her completely into his confidence and told her, "No razor has touched my head, for I have been consecrated to God from my mother's womb. If I am shaved, my strength will leave me, and I shall be as weak as any other man." When Delilah saw that he had taken her completely into his confidence, she summoned the lords of the Philistines, saying, "Come up this time, for he has opened his heart to me." So the lords of the Philistines came and brought up the money with them. She had him sleep on her lap, and called for a man who shaved off his seven locks of hair. Then she began to mistreat him, for his strength had left him. When she said, "The Philistines are upon you, Samson!" and he woke from his sleep, he thought he could make good his escape as he had done time and again, for he did not realize that the LORD had left him.

Ehret points our attention to these Bible verses, as they show how the power and vitality of a strong human was lost as soon as they shaved or cut their hair. For Ehret and many of his Back-to-naturist peers, the shaving and cutting of one's hair is not only unnatural, but debilitating and unhealthy. From this perspective, the ability to grow one's hair is a sign of cleanliness and superior health.

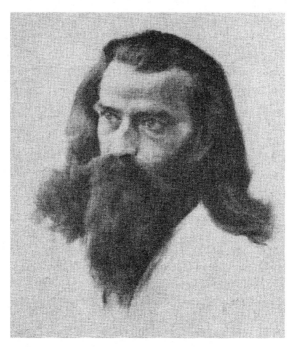

Sketch of a photo of Ehret taken after a 40-day fast that shows a great amount of facial and longer head hair.

Sex—Part 2

Lesson XXIV

Motherhood and Eugenics[103]

Motherhood with a mucusless diet, before, during, and after pregnancy is the development towards the Madonna-like, holy purity principal different from the dangerous, so-called "ordinary" childbirth, with its ever-present risk of life, known in our present civilization.

If the female body is perfectly clean through this diet, the menstruation disappears. In scriptures, it is called by the significant word "purification," which it in fact is. It is clean and no longer polluted by the monthly flow of impure blood and other wastes. This is the ideal condition of an inside purity capable of "immaculate conception." When seen in the light of this truth, the entire "Madonna mystery" is easily understood.

Every one of my female patients reported their menses as becoming less and less, then a 2-, 3-, and 4-month intermission, and finally entirely disappearing. The latter condition was experienced by those who went through a perfect cleansing process by this diet.

Headaches, toothaches, vomiting, and all other so-called "diseases of pregnancy" disappear. This leads to painless childbirth, an ample sufficiency of very sweet milk, babies that never cry, babies who are

179

very differently "clean," as compared with others, are the wonderful facts I have learned from every woman becoming a mother after having lived on this diet.

It is not advisable to start a radical change in diet during pregnancy, or while nursing; this should be done at least 2 or 3 months before conception.

"Eating for two," with a special diet is unnecessary if the body is clean. Modern babies are overfed, hence these dangerous childbirths. The only reasonable change is to increase the eating of natural sweets such as figs, raisins, dates, grapes, etc.

Feeding the Baby

If mother's milk is found to be insufficient or bad, do not use plain cow's milk. It should be diluted with at least one-third to one-half water and sweetened with milk sugar or honey. Start feeding the baby as soon as possible with a teaspoonful of good fruit juices (juice from stewed beets is also good) and honey diluted in water between meals. The baby's craving is sweet, and proves that fruit sugar is the "essence" of all dietetics.

What is considered a well-fed and healthy looking baby, of average normal weight, is in reality pounds of waste or decayed milk.

Whether the baby is sick or not, as soon as you commence feeding it fruit juices and stewed mash fruits, you will learn from the elimination that I am correct. The change must therefore be made very carefully. Babies and children must go through the same cleansing, healing process as do adults. I believe that a baby well nursed by good mother's milk on this diet and without "special" protein foods will grow wonderfully, and after the weaning period is over could be raised on apples alone.

As stated before, if a change of this kind in the baby's diet is made, they must be healed first—whether sick or not—cleansed from the waste of their "latent disease." This is the point that everyone refuses to believe, realize, or understand.

Natural sweets are necessary for the growing child for building a strong skeleton. Lime is also important.

I learned through the few examples that we had in Europe, that the character, the mind in general of the growing child, is greatly and beneficially influenced by this diet, with the progress of the purity of the body. The "troubles" of raising children from which you can be saved are enormous. No more children's diseases!

Thousands of mothers, unconsciously through overeating, practically kill their children before they are born. Here then is the only and correct way to fight infantile mortality. *There is no higher moral duty of any kind than to produce a perfect being.*

Eugenics of a Diseaseless, Superior Race

Using a plant as a comparison, "motherhood" can be said to represent the QUALITY of the soil; "fatherhood" represents the quality of the seed—of the germ.

A relatively poor, almost barren soil but a good quality of seed produces a fairly good plant, but a *defective* seed, even though planted in the best soil, will produce NOTHING.

Breeders of animals, especially horse breeders, know that the quality of a thoroughbred father goes through endless generations, even spanning over a chain of "indifferent" mothers. This is why inheritance of good and bad qualities (tuberculosis for instance) skips a whole generation.

As in every aspect of life, this problem is different also, and, of course, is different in the case of a clean body on a natural diet. Medical doctors and naturopaths alike will hardly believe at all in the new principles and arguments which I have brought out and postulated in this work. They reason and argue with the facts and experiences of the filthy body living on the unnatural diet of civilization.

You cannot reason about colors with a person born blind. You cannot use the old arguments and the old physiology to refute my statements.

Until you have personally experienced on your own body the truth of my teachings, you will have to accept and believe the new ones.

Realize, please, what this means—SUPERIOR FASTINGS—as they were taken by the prophets of old.

During a period covering some decades, and even partly today, the science of eugenics believed in the necessity of outside breeding. They consider outside breeding an absolute necessity for animals and the human race based on the bad results which accrued from the inbreeding of humans.

It is nothing less than the problem of the future of the American Nation—mixing races or inbreeding? The Jewish race is the answer. It is the only in existence where inbreeding is natural and perfect. Marriage of close relationship fails simply because we have degenerated too far, in comparison with the people of their ancestor Abraham. Outside breeding is a "stimulation" with an apparently good result, lasting only for one or two generations and then, in general, the family dies out.

The European royal family kept their genealogical tree clean, securing good results only so long as they did not live in modern luxury. The families of noblemen are rapidly disappearing because they failed to continue the generation of males. The luxurious diet of today, instead of the old-fashioned simplicity of centuries ago, is to blame. Former generations lived as farmers (a more natural life). Today they are the typical "high livers" in modern Sodoms; no wonder an expiring degeneration is the result!

Predetermination of Sex

What I will endeavor to show here is how to produce a genius, and this will prove at the same time that the predetermination of the sex is based on a higher principle than on the time of conception only.

Again and again, diet is everything. Humans are what they eat! Are not all geniuses, great men, inventors, the greatest artists of every kind born of poor parentage!

182

Why did the birth of male babies increase during the European war? They will become good and intelligent men. Restriction in diet and restriction in sexual intercourse—that is all! The cleaner the body of both parents, the less frequent the intercourse, the smaller the quantity of good food, the greater the love vibrations become, and with these conditions the better the chance for a genius, and that is always a boy. The most ideal example of this truth, and it is said to be a historical fact, is this:

During the black plague centuries ago, a number of young people took refuge together in a house in the neighborhood of Florence, Italy. For weeks they had nothing to eat and then, of course, only sparsely. They became married and generated the family of the Medici, which produced the greatest statesmen, artists, and scientists of every kind known in the history of western civilization.

We know that vitality vibrates through a waste-free body more perfectly than one encumbered with food. This is the superior fast with its indescribable conditions. Yet more difficult of description are love vibrations—when humans ascend to a God-like being, as they must have been in prehistoric times on the divine diet. The magnetic sex emanations become so wonderful that love combined with gluttony appears as a crime.

For the young couple to fast on their wedding day is a Jewish religious custom, but it is only a reminder of a hygienic law of that great statesman Moses—to generate geniuses through superior waves of love through the infinite.

It is the principle by which the male stock, when living on "clean" food, has the opportunity to generate a diseaseless, superior one.

Everyone who travels a little further upwards on the road towards the "paradise-like" conditions of humans will soon sense this truth. Humans were once a higher, superior kind of being, not a species of the monkey family![104] We are only a shade of the original human, caused through our degeneration, but you may yet experience what cannot be described, that this kind of eugenics is the fundamental truth of evolution into "Heaven on Earth!"

183

[103] The term *eugenics* was coined in 1883, along with the adjective *eugenic*, by English scientist Francis Galton (1822-1911). It is an analogy of ethics, physics, etc. from Greek *eugenes* or "well-born, of good stock, of noble race," from *eu-* "good" + *genos* "birth." The term is associated with a biosocial movement and philosophy advocating the improvement of human hereditary traits through promoting higher reproduction of more desired people and traits, and reduced reproduction of less desired people and traits. Propagators tended to believe in the genetic superiority of Nordic, Germanic, and Anglo-Saxon peoples; supported strict immigration and anti-miscegenation laws; and supported forcible sterilization of the poor, disabled, and "immoral."

Ehret uses the term "eugenics" to make a philosophical point about the potential for developing an improved race of humans through the *Mucusless Diet Healing System*. For many modern readers, this term is off-putting due to its historic association with racist and genocidal policies. Of course, Ehret wrote this text well before the climax of radical eugenic policies in the United States and by Aldof Hitler in Germany. Yet, Ehret's beliefs about a so-called superior race of people are diametrically opposed to the white supremacist mentality that was the foundation of most eugenic programs. Ehret's proposition is that what we identify to be race, which is accepted today as a socially constructed belief system and not a biological fact by most scientists and academics, is a physical expression of the degree to which one's organism is overcome by mucus/toxemias. In other words, the darker you are, the more mucusless you are. This perspective is in line with scientific findings that reveal Homo sapiens to be a tropical, frugivorous (fruit-eating) species that has its origins in equatorial Africa. Ehret is not using the term in a bigoted way, insofar as he proudly speaks of his skin becoming darker while doing long fruit fasts. On the other hand, he says that he noticed that his skin became lighter after eating even one piece of bread. Thus, from Ehret's perspective, skin color is not based upon how close an organism lives to the equator, or on the production of melanin (what Ehret refers to as "mineral salts"), but is based primarily on the amount of uneliminated waste the body contains on the cellular level.

In sum, Ehret's use of the word eugenics is quite unique and different from many of his peers. Today, terms such as genetics, natural selection, evolution, etc., may be more politically correct labels to make the kind of points Ehret is espousing. Essentially, it is a "survival of the fittest" argument, whereby the fittest humans are those that live in accordance with natural laws and eat a mucusless diet.

[104] This is quite a profound statement by Ehret. In these latter chapters, he tends to reveal some of his more metaphysical and spiritual philosophies. Here, Ehret rejects the notion of Darwinian evolution (that humans evolved from the ape family) and suggests that the origin of humans comes from a higher plane. Perhaps humans degenerated from a source that had no beginning and no ending. Many followers of Ehret also reject the theory of evolution and have adopted a theory of "devolution" whereby humans are actively eating themselves downward deeper into the animal kingdom. For more on these concepts, see *Spira Speaks: Dialogs and Essays on the Mucusless Diet Healing System.*

The Enforcement of Elimination by Physical Adjustments:

Exercises, Sunbaths, Internal Baths, and Bathing

Lesson XXV

As shown in previous lessons, all physical treatments vibrate or shake the tissues and thereby stimulate the circulation in one way or another for the purpose and with the result of loosening and eliminating "foreign matters," the cause of all diseases.[105] The human body does this itself, in the most perfect way, as soon as you fast or as soon as your blood composition has been changed by natural diet.

Physical treatments and physical culture can therefore be combined with this diet and fasting to enforce and to hasten the elimination. However, I must advise that extreme care be taken not to exaggerate, especially on "bad" days—days of strong elimination. If you are tired and you feel bad, then rest and sleep just as much as you can. On the days that you feel "good" during a fast or strict diet, you may take some physical treatment also, such as exercise, baths, massage, deep breathing, etc.

The most natural exercises, and by far the best, are walking, dancing, and singing. The latter is the most natural breathing exercise with the added advantage of loosening by chest vibrations.[106] An excellent "exercise," and one that everybody knows, is hiking in the mountains. When climbing hills, you increase your breathing in the most natural way. Your breathing becomes better and more harmoniously than with any "system" of exercises.

The cleaner you become the more easily you will understand what I teach in Lesson V—that air and the other ingredients of the forests are "food"—invisible food.

Both hands should be free when walking, so as to permit continually the natural movements.

Outdoor garden work is another natural exercise.

By taking proper care of your body, you will generate health. The following exercises are suggested for those who desire to keep physically fit. I must again remind you that air is more necessary to life than food. Proper breathing is therefore essential. *Do not exercise in a close, stuffy room.* Stand before an open window. Take a deep, full breath with each exercise. Inhale through nose and expel through mouth. Stand before a mirror while exercising, and admire the suppleness and graceful manner in which you perform each movement. Fall in love with yourself if no one else will. Keep the feet about 15 inches apart—stand erect and use muscular tension.

Exercise No. 1

Standing erect, hands to the side, clench the fists tightly. Raise arms slowly as high above the head as possible, taking a deep breath. Relax and expel breath. Repeat five times.

Exercise No. 2

Extend arms and ensure that your arms are at your chest level. Grasp hands tightly and pull to the right side, resisting with left hand. Then go through same motion pulling to the left side. Relax after each motion, expelling breath. Repeat each exercise five times.

Exercise No. 3

Grasp the left hand firmly with the right, in front of body. Resisting with the left hand, lift with the right, using full strength while raising the arms high above your head. Take a deep breath on the upward motion, and relax before expelling. Repeat with the right hand resisting with the left, five times each.

Exercise No. 4

Clasp hands above the head, allowing them to rest on your head. Bend to the right side, pulling hard, then to the left five times, and then alternate first right and then left. Between each movement take a deep breath and expel when relaxed. This exercise is especially good for stimulating the liver.

Exercise No. 5

Clasp hands in back of neck, holding all muscles tense. Twist to the right, then to the left five times. Now pull to the right and then to the left five times. Now pull to the left and then to the right five times. Hold your legs rigid, but permit your body to sway.

Exercise No. 6

Grasp the hands behind the back and without bending the body, raise arms up as far as possible. Inhale on the upward motion; relax and expel. Repeat five times. This exercise is for developing the chest.

Exercise No. 7

Place your right hand over your right hip, clench left fist, and raise left arm slowly, taking a deep breath. At the same time, bend the body as far to the right as possible. Make it hurt. Relax and expel breath. Repeat with left hand placed on hip, and raise right arm with fist tightly clenched. Repeat each five times.

Exercise No. 8

Grasp hands firmly in front of breast, all muscles tense; and twist to the left. Now twist to the right as far as possible. Do not permit feet to move. Inhale during motion; relax and expel breath. Repeat each exercise five times.

Exercise No. 9

Raise arms above the head as high as possible, even permitting body to bend backwards. Now bend body forwards and without bending the knees try to touch the floor with your fingers. Exhale breath when relaxed. Repeat this exercise slowly five times, and gradually increase to 20 times.

189

Do not exhaust yourself in any of the exercises. If the exercises make you stiff at first, it is a sure sign that you needed them, and that they are doing you good. The soreness will soon wear off if you continue the exercises persistently. You may add other exercises to these, but be sure they have the deep breathing. *Play your favorite music when exercising.* Any snappy march piece will do.[107] The vibrations from the music are wonderful. It is preferable to exercise the first thing in the morning—immediately upon arising. If clothing is worn, it should be loose. Start with a few exercises at first and then increase gradually. Above all things, do not consider it a duty, but put fun into them. Dancing alone and bending movements to the accompaniment of music will prove very beneficial.

Sunbaths

Whenever you have an opportunity of doing so, take a sunbath. In the beginning, do not exceed 20 to 30 minutes and keep the head covered. On "bad" days—days of great elimination—stay cool.

The cleaner you become, the more you will enjoy the sunbath and the longer you will remain. You will also find that you can stand it much warmer. A short cool shower or a cool rub with a towel dampened in cold water immediately after the sunbath is good.

The sunbath is an excellent "invisible" waste eliminator, and it rejuvenates the skin, causing it to become silk-like and coloring it a natural brown. Civilized men and women of our race show by their white skin that they are sick from birth on; they inherit the mucused, white blood corpuscles—the "sign of death."

As all of the clothing should be removed during a sunbath, a small enclosure just long enough to lie in should be built in your backyard, or even on the roof, away from prying, inquisitive eyes. The clothing of civilization has made it impossible for humans to secure their proper quota of the life-giving power of fresh air and sunshine, so essential to health and happiness. The direct rays of the sun on the naked body supply the electricity, energy, and vitality to the human storage battery, renewing it in vigor, strength, and virility.[108]

Internal Baths

During the transition period, even though you have regular bowel movements, *it is advisable to wash out the lower colon.* The sticky waste, slimy mucus, and various poisons which Nature is attempting to eject should be helped along as much as possible. A small-bulb infant syringe can be used after the regular bowel movement, but for a thorough cleansing, two to three quarts of water should be used.[109]

Try to have a natural bowel movement before injecting the water. The body should be in a reclining position, lying on the right side.[110] The syringe must not be higher than three or four feet above the patient. Water should be warm, not hot, and it should be tested on your elbow. Should any discomfort be felt, stop the flow until the discomfort passes as the entire two or three quarts should be retained at one time. If the cramp or pain becomes too great, allow the water to pass from the colon and repeat the operation.

The water should remain in the intestines for about 15 or 20 minutes, or as long as it is comfortable. While still lying on your side, gently massage the colon in an upward motion. Then lie on the back with the knees drawn up and massage from right side of body to left; now turn over, lying on the left side, and massage the left side with a downward motion. You should now be ready for ejecting the water. The best time to take an enema is just before retiring.

Bathing

Authorities differ on bathing almost as widely as they do on diet. The *Mucusless Diet Healing System* will produce the "skin you love to touch" through clean blood supply, and without the aid of cosmetics, lotions, and cold creams.

It is not necessary to take a daily hot bath with soap and brush under ordinary conditions.

The morning "cold shower" during the entire year, without any consideration of weather conditions is also inadvisable. There is no need to deliberately subject the body to an extreme shock, and in a number of cases more harm than good may result.

191

Needless to state, the skin must be kept clean so that the pores may be permitted to properly function, and this can be accomplished by the following method:

Place a basin of cool water before you. Dip the hands in the basin and starting with the face, rub briskly; wet the hands again and apply to the neck and shoulders; next rub the chest and stomach; next the arms and then the back, and last the legs and feet. Put the feet right into the basin if you care to. Keep moistening the hands as needed, but there is no necessity for throwing any quantity of water on the body. To dry off, rub with the bare hands for 5 minutes, if possible until the body is all aglow, or wipe with a towel. This should be done upon arising immediately after you have taken your exercises. The results will surprise you. If you prefer a tub bath, then allow about one inch of cold water to run into the tub. Sit in it with knees drawn up, and follow the same rule of rubbing and massage as outlined above.

Remember that the air bath is just as essential as the water bath. A few minutes each day spent before an open window, upon arising and just before retiring, when all clothes are removed, massaging the body—help the skin to retain its natural functioning qualities.[111]

Always bear in mind that extremes of any kind are harmful. This applies to exercise, bathing, and sleeping, as well as extremes in eating. Even extreme joy and happiness has been known to kill just as readily as extreme anger, hate, and worry. Therefore, AVOID EXTREMES OF ALL KINDS.

---

[105] Ehret does not advocate excessive exercise for the purposes of loosening and eliminating waste. Historically, there have been various therapies that use intensive shaking and massage as a primary means to loosen waste. For Ehret, rational and natural physical activity is best, and excessive exercise and massage should be avoided.

[106] Practicing the "Science of Breath" or rational forms of yoga go hand-in-hand with the mucusless diet.

[107] Feel free to listen to something other than marches if you are moved to do so. Historically, marches became one of the most popular forms of

music around the world throughout the 1800s and early 1900s. Before the advent of phonograph records, if people wanted to hear music they had to either make it themselves or see it performed live. The military band craze of the 1800s is even partly responsible for the marching bands that still play a visible role in school and university music programs. With that said, Ehret was a man of his times, and the prospect of exercising to a phonograph record was innovative and exciting.

[108] The power of sunbathing to aid the body in cleansing must not be underestimated. It is recommended to not use sun-blocking lotions which terribly constipate the pores. As with all aspects of the diet, be sure to transition into longer periods in the sun. The cleaner you become, the easier it will be to safely and naturally lavish in the hot sun for long periods of time.

[109] Two or three quarts of water is the amount that fits in most standard enema bags. Many modern-day mucusless diet practitioners use lemon juice and distilled water enemas regularly. For more details about doing enemas, see the section on lemon juice enemas in *Spira Speaks: Dialogs and Essays on the Mucusless Diet Healing System*.

[110] There are different schools of thought about what is best to lie on. For a more detailed discussion about this see the lemon enema section in *Spira Speaks: Dialogs and Essays on the Mucusless Diet Healing System*.

[111] A good rule of thumb is to not put anything on your skin that you would not be prepared to eat. Soap, makeup, lotions, deodorant, etc., all enter your body through your pores. It is recommended to find soaps, etc., made with the most natural ingredients. Many supermarkets now carry natural hygiene products in their "organic" or "natural" foods sections. It is strongly recommended that you avoid using standard deodorants, which terribly clog up the pores of your underarms. Armpit odor comes from one of two sources: 1) the stench of internal wastes, or 2) bacteria tucked away in the outside of your pits. The former source radically decreases as you cleanse your insides of putrid waste. For the latter, I've found **lemon juice underarm air baths** to be the greatest way to safely eliminate foul odor from the outside of the body. Juice one lemon, then take a clean cloth or paper towel (all natural with no inks is preferable) and sop up some of the juice. Then apply it to your underarms, one at a time. Afterwards, raise your arms toward the sky for several minutes and let the lemon juice air dry. Letting the oxygen dry the juice helps to eliminate all odor causing agents.

This method can be much cheaper and less harmful than using store-bought deodorants or antiperspirants.

(Many mucusless diet practitioners buy lemons, and other items, in bulk from local grocers or fruit and vegetable wholesalers. Wholesalers often have "cash-and-carry" options and will be willing to sell you boxes of fruits and vegetables for the whole family.)

A Message to Ehretists

Dear Friends:

After careful and intelligent study of the foregoing lessons, you now know that disease consists of an unknown, decayed, and fermented mass of matter in the human body, decades old—especially in the intestines and colon. You likewise know how unwise and ignorant it is to think that knowing what to eat is, alone, a complete diet of healing.

None of the recognized authorities know the tremendous importance of a thorough and deep cleansing of the human "cesspool." All are more or less "fooled" by nature when they advise eating of fruits, with stomach and intestines clogged up by mucus and decomposed protein foods, eaten from childhood onwards right into adulthood and beyond.

You have been taught the result: should these poisons—cyanide of potassium—be dissolved too rapidly and permitted to enter the circulation, severe sensations—even death—may occur, and human's natural food, oranges, grapes, dates, etc., are blamed!

My teachings clearly prove that this hitherto unexplained ignorance regarding fruit diet is the "stumbling-block" for all other food research experts, who have made personal experimental tests. I have heard the same cry thousands of times and even from young and supposedly healthy persons—"I became weak!" And all experts,

195

with the exception of me, say "Yes, you require more protein; at least eat nuts."

During my personal tests involving this same problem, I tried to overcome this "stumbling-block" hundreds of times. After a 2-year cure in Italy of Bright's disease with consumptive tendency, by fasting and strict living on a mucusless diet, I ate two pounds of the sweetest grapes and drank half a gallon of fresh, sweet grape juice, made from the best and most wonderful grapes grown there. Almost immediately, I felt as though I were going to die! A terrible sensation overcame me, palpitation of the heart, extreme dizziness which forced me to lie down, and I was seized with severe pains in the stomach and intestines. After 10 minutes, the great event occurred— a mucus-foaming diarrhea and vomiting of grape juice mixed with acid-smelling mucus, and then the greatest event of all! I felt so wonderfully well and strong that I at once performed the knee-bending and arm-stretching exercises 326 times consecutively. All obstructions had been removed!

For the first time in history, I have shown what humans were when they lived without "fired" foods—during the prehistoric times (called Paradise) eating fruits, the "bread of heaven."

For the first time in human history this "demon" in the tragedy of human life has been shown—and how they can and must be eliminated—before men and women can again ascend to a Paradisiacal health, happiness, immunity from disease and "God-like" being.

If the Garden of Eden—heaven on earth—ever existed it must have been a "fruit orchard." For thousands of years, through wrong civilization, humans have been tricked into unconscious suicide, reduced to slavery, to produce wrong food, "earning their bread by the sweat of their brow." Unnatural foods cause sickness and death.

"Peace on Earth" happiness and righteousness as yet remain a foolish dream. During thousands of years, God, Paradise, Heaven— Sin, Devil, Hell—seldom found an interpretation that a clear, reasoning mind would willingly accept. The average unfortunate fellowman thinks of God as a good and forgiving Father who will allow him to enter Paradise in another world—unpunished for any violations of His laws in nature.

I have proven for the first time in history that the diet of Paradise is not only possible—good enough for degenerate humankind, such as we now are—but that it is the Unconditional Necessity and the first step to real salvation and redemption from the misery of life. That it is a needed key to the lost paradise where disease, worry, and sorrow—hate, fight, and murder—were unknown, and where there was no death, from unnatural causes at least.

"We are what we eat" is a philosopher's greatest and truest statement.

You must now see why civilization, all religion, all philosophy, with their tremendous sacrifice of work, time, money, energy, is and has been part guesswork. The magic formula for "Heaven on Earth"—of the Paradise—must read like this:

"Eat your way into Paradise physically." But you cannot pass the gate, watched over by the angel with the flaming sword, until you have gone through purgatory (cleansing fire) of fasting and diet of healing—a cleansing, a physiological purifying, by the "Flame of Life" in your own body! For thousands of years no one has escaped the struggle of death caused by an unnatural life, and you will have to face it someday.

But you, I, and others who have learned this greatest and most important truth of life, are the only ones in existence today who are in fact, and not by mind only, out of the road of darkness and unconscious suicide and into the light of the new civilization—the light of a physical regeneration—as the foundation of mental and spiritual revelation-like progress to the light of a superior, that is to say, a spiritual world.

This book represents an outline of the serious nature of my work and it also appeals to you for help in carrying it through as the greatest deed you can perform—upon which depends not only your future destiny, but that of a suffering, unhappy humankind—on the verge of physical and mental collapse.

ARNOLD EHRET

INDEX

D

E

F

fruitarian, 15, 170, 172

G

geniuses, 182
goiter, 30
gonorrhea, 173–74
gout, 30, 86, 168
Graham, Rev. Sylvester, 86, 89
grains, 13, 57, 100, 103, 117

H

Haig, Dr. Alexander, 23, 25, 85–86
hair, health of, 176, 177, 178
Hensel, Dr. Julius, 47, 50, 67, 69, 86
herbs, medicinal, 116, 118–19
how to break, 143

I

impotence, 176
indigestion, 22, 36
influenza, 18, 41
innerclean. *See* "intestinal broom, herbal", *See* "intestinal broom, herbal"
intestinal broom
  herbal, 3, 116
  vegetable, 86, 113, 122

J

Jaeger, Dr. Gustav, 23, 25

K

Kellogg, Dr. John Harvey, 55, 56
kidney diseases, 30, 157

L

Lahmann, Dr. Johann Heinrich, 23, 25, 85, 86, 95
legumes, 103, 167

liver diseases, 30
lungs, 18, 29, 32, 46, 54

M

magic mirror, 35–43, 83, 167–68
massage, 76, 187, 191
masturbation, 176
meats, 13, 166
medicine, 22, 25, 38, 54–55, 62, 75–76, 80
menstruation, 179
mental Diseases, 31
mental Treatments, 76, 77, 78
metabolism, 53, 54, 55, 56, 57, 72
milk, 26, 40, 60, 62, 66, 72, 85, 100, 166, 179
milk diet, 88
mineral salts, 66, 73, 86, 123–24, 165, 167, 184
motherhood, 179, 180, 181
mucus-lean diet, 112, 115, 122–24, 127, 140

N

naturopathy, 3, 10, 14, 22, 23, 35, 38, 42, 46, 59, 88, 174

P

physiology, the new, 10, 46, 53–74, 161, 169
Powell, Dr. Thomas, 65–67, 68–69

R

raw food, 91, 92, 95, 123, 130
raw food diet. *See* raw food
raw foodism. *See* row food

S

sex
  diseases, 30, 173
  natural control of, 175–76
  psychology, 175
stammering, 30, 32

standard combination salad, 113
starch, 10, 27, 37, 61, 65, 67, 86, 87, 97, 129
sterility, 176
syphilis, 33, 173

T

toothaches, 29, 179
transition diet, 90, 111–40

U

uneliminated, 9, 36

V

V equals P minus O (V = P - O), 45–50
vegan, 103
veganism. *See* vegan
vegetarian, 4, 6, 55, 60, 85, 86, 103, 129, 130, 138, 140, 145, 149
Venereal Diseases, 33, 149, 173

W

water fasting, 157, 162
water fasts. *See* water fasting

ABOUT PROF. SPIRA

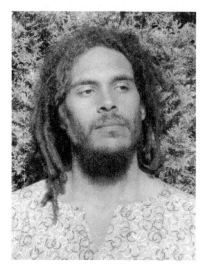

In 2002, Prof. Spira was a 280-pound former high school football player suffering from multiple ailments such as daily migraine headaches, allergies, regular bouts of bronchitis, sleep apnea, persistent heartburn, etc. After having lost his mother to a terrible string of chronic illnesses when he was in the 6th grade, he grew up assuming that he was genetically destined to be sick his whole life. While studying jazz trombone performance at the University of Cincinnati's College Conservatory of Music, he met a jazz drummer named Willie Smart (aka Brother Air) who told him about Arnold Ehret's *Mucusless Diet Healing System*. Within 6 months of reading the book, Spira lost 110 pounds and overcame all of his major ailments. He was able to throw away his CPAP unit (an oxygen mask that treats sleep apnea) and the medications he'd taken since childhood. Since his transformation, Spira has helped and inspired numerous people to use the mucusless diet to overcome their illnesses through his writings, music, and one-on-one consultations.

Spira is a professional jazz trombonist, educator, and author. He holds an MM in jazz trombone performance, an MA in African American and African Studies, and is a Ph.D. candidate in ethnomusicology at the Ohio State University. He is also the co-leader of an all-vegetarian and Ehretist jazz group entitled the Breathairean Ensemble, whose members are dedicated to inspiring their listeners to pursue what they call "physiological liberation." In 2013, Spira published his first book about the mucusless diet entitled *Spira Speaks: Dialogs and Essays on the Mucusless Diet Healing System*. He is the webmaster of www.mucusfreelife.com.

Spira Speaks: Dialogs and Essays on the
Mucusless Diet Healing System

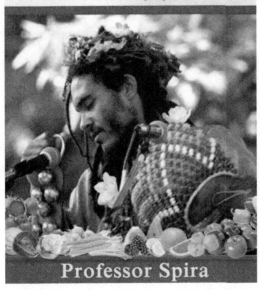

Join Prof. Spira for an unprecedented look into the healing power of a mucus-free lifestyle! After losing 110 pounds and overcoming numerous physical ailments, Spira learned that he had a gift for articulating the principles of the diet through writing and music. As he began to interact with health-seekers on the internet in 2005, he realized that written dialogs about the diet could benefit far more than just its intended readers. This book is a compilation of the best writings by Professor Spira on the subject.

What is the *Mucusless Diet Healing System*? How has it helped numerous people overcome illnesses thought to be permanent? What does it take to practice a mucus-free lifestyle in the twenty-first century? Why is the transition diet one of the most misunderstood aspects of the mucusless diet? Spira answers these questions and much more in his unprecedented new book that contains never-before released writings about the mucusless diet.

Pamphlets on Ehret's Teachings

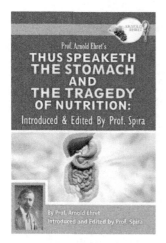
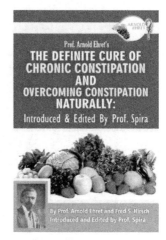

Thus Speaketh the Stomach and A Tragedy of Nutrition

If your intestines could talk, what would they say? What if you could understand health through the perspective of your stomach? In this unprecedented work, Arnold Ehret gives voice to the stomach and reveals the foundation of human illness.

The Definite Cure of Chronic Constipation and Overcoming Constipation Naturally: Introduction by Prof. Spira

In the Definite Cure of Chronic Constipation and Overcoming Constipation Naturally, Prof. Arnold Ehret and his number-one student Fred Hirsch explore generally constipated condition of the human organism.

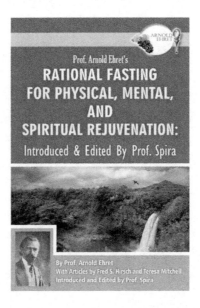

Discover one of Ehret's most vital and influential works, and companion to the *Mucusless Diet Healing System*. Introducing *Rational Fasting for Physical, Mental, and Spiritual Rejuvenation: Introduced and Edited by Prof. Spira*, now available from Breathair Publishing.

In this masterpiece, Ehret explains how to successfully, safely, and rationally conduct a fast in order to eliminate harmful waste from the body and promote internal healing. Also included are famous essays on Ehret's teachings by Fred Hirsch and long-time devotee Teresa Mitchell.

You will learn:

- The Common Fundamental Cause in the Nature of Diseases
- Complete Instructions for Fasting
- Building a Perfect Body through Fasting
- Important Rules for the Faster
- How Long to Fast
- Why to Fast
- When and How to Fast
- How Teresa Mitchell Transformed Her Life through Fasting
- And Much More!

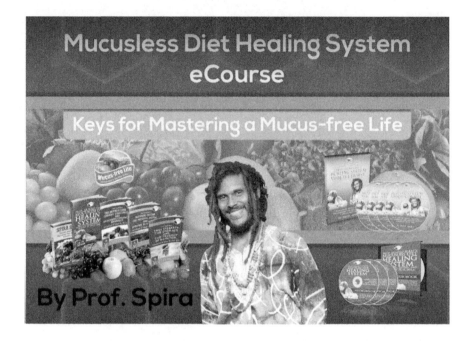

In this unprecedented six weeklong intensive online course, you will learn everything that you need to know about Arnold Ehret's *Mucusless Diet Healing System*, and how to get started on the path toward a Mucus-free Lifestyle.

The Art of Transition: Spira's
Mucusless Diet Healing System Menu and Recipe Guide

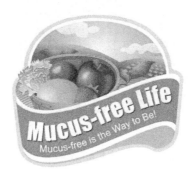

What does a mucusless diet practitioner actually eat? What kind of transitional mucus-forming foods are best? What are the most effective menu combinations to achieve long-lasting success with the mucusless diet? What are the best transitional cooked and raw menus? What foods and combinations should be avoided at all costs? How can you prepare satisfying mucusless and mucus-lean meals for your family?

These questions and much more will be addressed in Prof. Spira's long-awaited mucusless diet menu and recipe book! Stay tuned!

Introduction, Purpose, Popular Fruits, Vegetables, and Vegan Items Omitted from this Book, Organic vs. Non-organic, Mucus-lean, Raw vs. Cooked, Satisfying Nut and Dried Fruit Combinations, The Onion Sauté, Filling Steamed and Baked Vegetable Meals, Spira's Special "Meat-Away" Meal, Mucusless, Raw Combination Salads, Raw Dressings, Favorite Mono-fruit Meals, Favorite Dried Fruits, Favorite Fruit Combinations, Vegetable Juices, Fruit Smoothies and Sauces, Fresh Fruit Juices, Sample Combinations and Weekly Menus

Projected Release: Winter 2015

SPIRA'S MUCUSLESS DIET
COACHING & CONSULTATIONS

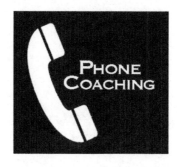

After receiving a consultation with Professor Spira, I was able to take my practice of the Mucusless Diet Healing System to a new level. Speaking face to face with an advanced practitioner was key and a true blessing on my journey. I'm looking forward to following up with another in the future!

-Brian Stern, Certified Bikram Yoga Instructor and Musician

You truly are amazing. You have done nothing but given all you can to help me and I truly appreciate this. Thank you for "feeding me."

-Samantha Claire, Pianist and Educator

Spira has practiced the mucusless diet and studied the natural hygienic/back-to-nature movements for the past 13 years. During that time, he has advised and helped many in the art of transitioning away from mucus-forming foods. For a limited time, talk with Prof. Spira about your individual needs, challenges, and questions. Skype, telephone, or in-person consultations available! For more information, visit:

www.mucusfreelife.com/diet-coaching

WEB LINKS

Websites

mucusfreelife.com

breathairmusic.com

Facebook

Prof. Spira Fan Page: www.facebook.com/ProfessorSpira

Arnold Ehret Fan Page: www.facebook.com/arnoldehret.us

Arnold Ehret Support Group: www.facebook.com/groups/arnoldehret/

YouTube

Prof. Spira's Breathair-Vision: www.youtube.com/user/professorspira

Twitter

@profspira

@ArnoldEhret1

Visit our Bookstore to Find Books by Arnold Ehret!

www.mucusfreelife.com/storefront/

Spira is now available for mucusless diet consultations/coaching!

www.mucusfreelife.com/mucusless-coaching/

Please Share Your Reviews!

Share your reviews and comments about this book and your experiences with the mucusless diet on Amazon and mucusfreelife.com. Prof. Spira would love to hear how the text has helped you.

PEACE, LOVE, AND BREATH!

Printed in Great Britain
by Amazon